IN A LEAGUE
OF THEIR OWN

The story of the Women's League of
Health and Beauty

Lynn Ashburner

Foreword by Prunella Stack

Published by Heritage Books

PUBLISHED BY:

Heritage Books
34 Mucklestone Rd
Loggerheads
Market Drayton
TF9 4ES

PRINTED BY:

Sherwin Rivers Ltd
Waterloo Road
Cobridge
Stoke on Trent
ST6 3HR

ISBN:

0-9549963-0-5

ACKNOWLEDGEMENTS:

My very sincere thanks to everyone at the League who has given of their time: Prunella Stack, Margaret Peggie, Terri Adams, Peter Hobden and Council members.

A special thanks to those who agreed to be interviewed: current members, trainers and organisers, who have told me their stories and shared their memories:

> Rosemary Barber, Peggy Bold, Carol Bentley, Marjorie Challenor, Pat Edwards, Joyce Ellison, Barbara Furniss, Shirley Gaitley, Fiona Gillanders, Sheila Gray, Doreen Handley, Valerie Higginson, Lucy Martin, Margaret McAllister, Marlene Morris, Sarah Price, Caroline Quigley, Margaret Sharpe, Brenda Toner, Betty Urquhart.

I am personally indebted to Margaret Peggie who made available to me her 1989 dissertation on the creation and development of the Women's League of Health and Beauty, and gave of her time freely, to help in the selection of photographs, to proof read and review the manuscript.

Grateful thanks to Prunella Stack for writing the Foreword and allowing me to quote from her two biographies. Mary Bagot Stack wrote 'Building the Body beautiful' in 1931. Prunella Stack and Mary's sister Norah Cruickshank, wrote a book about her life and work in 1937 'Movement is Life'. Prunella used the title 'Movement is Life' again for the book she wrote in 1973. This was followed by a biography of her mother, 'Zest for Life' in 1988.

THE AUTHOR

Lynn Ashburner is a professional writer and researcher living in Shropshire. She specialises in biography, oral history and organisational histories, and was previously an academic with many published books and articles. She also offers advice and help to anyone interested in writing their personal or family history.

This book is dedicated to the memory of Mary Bagot Stack and to all those who have carried forward her ideals - which have been an inspiration to thousands of women.

Proceeds from the sale of this book will go to future promotion of the League and the training of new teachers.

FOREWORD

In A League of Their Own is a history of the League's 75 years of existence. It provides a gamut of emotions – excitement, dedication, effort, belief, staying power and resolution, leading to rewards and fulfilment. The ups and downs of the League are like those of a life. Indeed it has been, in its own way, a chronicle of 70 years of the last century, and a brief 5 years of this one.

To the many who have helped its growth, and to whom it has presented a way of life, fitness and friendship, I give thanks – students, teachers, pianists, members, husbands, children and well-wishers! The vision in 1930 of our Founder, my mother Mary Bagot Stack, was the inspiration. This was followed by the excitement of a pioneer movement with youth's enthusiasm and nine years of spectacular growth. By 1939 the Membership had reached 150,000.

Then came the impact of stern reality – the War. The League kept going nevertheless, with 60 centres in being, and young teachers and members in the Forces or on war work. And when it ended, many of them returned to help rebuild the League. The Teacher Training School reopened and the League expanded once more.

A popular feature in the 70s and 80s was Elizabeth Mallett's trips to League centres abroad – Canada, South Africa, New Zealand – (and other delectable holiday spots!) These opened new horizons and encouraged new friendships.

The resumption of the Royal Albert Hall shows every five years, the continuity of Teacher Training, (the courses shortened and adapted to present day conditions), national recognition from the Fitness Council and links with similar movements, Medau and Keep Fit – all these served to enhance the League's life and position.

Now approaching its 75th birthday, the League has achieved a significant record of longevity! But I believe it is still young in heart, and hope it will always be so. Lynn Ashburner has chronicled all these events in her book. It will remind League members, and we hope the general public also, of a distinguished history. My thanks to her, and to all who have contributed to it, and best wishes for its success.

Prunella Stack
March 2005

IN A LEAGUE OF THEIR OWN

The story of the Women's League of Health and Beauty

CONTENTS

CHAPTER 1
SETTING THE SCENE

THE WOMEN'S LEAGUE OF HEALTH AND BEAUTY

The history of the Women's League of Health and Beauty is a fascinating story of how one woman's foresight and enthusiasm created a remarkable organisation that was both ahead of its time but also, of its time. Mary Bagot Stack born in 1883, in true pioneer fashion founded the Women's League of Health and Beauty in 1930, saw it flourish and grow to a membership of forty seven thousand by the time of her premature death less than five years later.

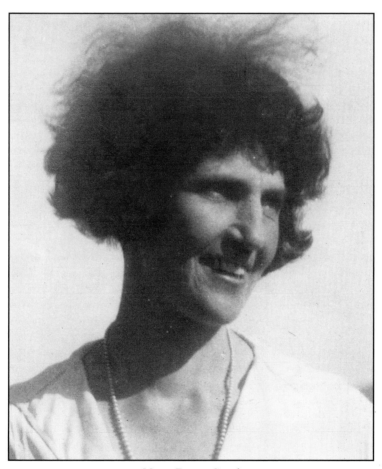

Mary Bagot Stack

This is the story of how Mary's dream became an international organisation that is now celebrating its seventy fifth birthday. It is not just a tribute to Mary, but to all her loyal friends, family and colleagues who ensured that her dream did not just live on but developed and maintained a relevance to women's lives across many decades. The story of the League is brought to life by the experiences of those who have been a part of the League and let the League become a part of their lives. These developments also need to be understood in relation to the important role it has modestly played in the social fabric of the country. As a movement created by and for women, it achieved success across all social strata, at a time when independence for women was far more limited than it is today.

SOCIAL CONTEXT

To fully comprehend Mary Bagot Stack's achievements there is a need to see them in the context of what it was like to be a woman in Britain in the early years of the last century. Although there were some changes in the lives of women there were also still many restrictions. 1900 to 1918 was the era that saw the birth of the suffragette movement with the rejection by many of the Victorian constraints on the behaviour and roles of women in society. It was signified by new fashions, with bobbed hair, short skirts, and the freedom to meet men without chaperones. The emancipation of women was a focal political issue, and the suffragette movement was soon thriving.

In 1914 there were about fifteen million women in Britain. Half were married or widowed and looking after homes and families, and ten per cent were single women working as housewives (unpaid). Another ten per cent worked as domestic servants or were in service. Less than four million women were employed outside the family, with many of these helping husbands or family to run a business rather than working independently. There are no records of the number of women entrepreneurs who began their own businesses or who forged ahead in their chosen career, as they formed only a small minority. This was not the role that was expected of women at this time. Any that chose to break taboos or challenge the status quo experienced strong resistance from many quarters, and those that succeeded did so in spite of this.

At the outbreak of the First World War about 400,000 women left domestic service to do other work and this contributed significantly to the 729,000 women who entered industry, replacing men who had gone to fight. Left to peacetime economic development, such an active role in all types of industry for women would not have happened for many decades. War made it a military and economic necessity. The primary roles for women during the war were as nurses, munitions workers and clerical labour. Others had to take on traditional male jobs on the factory floor. What is less commonly known is that as production lines were speeded up, all protective legislation was put aside, resulting in greater numbers of deaths and injuries.

After 1918 there was much to occupy politicians and the population in getting the country back to a more even keel. Returning troops needed to return to the workforce, and women who had so effectively taken their places, were required to vacate the positions they had held and to find alternative roles. Many women had thrived in their new and demanding roles, and did not wish to return to the type of work that they had had prior to 1914. Most significant was the unwillingness of women to return to domestic service. Alternative employment opportunities were emerging in the growth of clerical and office work, which although previously dominated by men, was beginning the process of becoming a predominantly female occupation.

This was also a time of increasing leisure for women and a loosening of social restraints. Young women were free to go out with friends of both sexes. Married women had greater access to contraception and as a consequence were having smaller families. The years between the wars also saw women's self help organisations develop. The suffragette movement had been a role model for women, however that was now in decline as partial emancipation had been established in 1918 with the vote given to women over thirty years of age subject to education and property rights. The vote was finally given to all women over the age of twenty one in 1928.

HEALTH AND EXERCISE

At the outset of the 21st century, we live in an age where leisure, health and exercise are an integral part of our lives, to a greater or lesser extent. We may assume that much of the current interest in fitness regimes and the phases of popularity of celebrity 'work-outs', aerobics, yoga, gym membership or pilates classes, are a relatively new phenomena. But as with so many ideas and fashions, nothing is ever quite as new as it seems. Early ideas are 'rediscovered' or re-emerge as 'new' with little or no acknowledgement to their past influences or inspiration. What most people, even those in the health and fitness industry, are unaware of, is that the origin of group exercise classes has a much longer and more interesting history. We have to go back to the early years of the last century to find the main precursors of today's exercise culture to be able to see the enduring extent of their influence. Whilst other European countries had well established organisations there was little happening in the UK, until Mary Bagot Stack took the initiative. Acknowledging the unique role played by the Women's League of Health and Beauty will add to our understanding of the history of exercise, health and fitness.

THE DEVELOPMENT OF EXERCISE

Many countries in the early 20th century developed an interest in exercise as a social activity, for the promotion of health and well being. Exercise movements across Europe fell into two main categories, those carried out for health and recreation, with altruistic and democratic aims, inviting people to join, and those that became associated with political, militaristic and non-democratic regimes. Two more marked opposites were hard to imagine. The latter became the most socially visible and are those that history has chosen to remember most vividly, despite their subsequent decline.

Between the wars there were several parallel developments. Scandinavia took the lead in the development of exercise across Europe and the Swedish Ling System was widely known in Britain. Per Hendrik Ling (1776-1839) had developed a series of free standing exercises which were performed without apparatus designed 'to correct or prevent bad posture and to cure faults of bodily development'. This included stretching exercises, lunging and exercises with a partner to provide support and resistance. These ideas were based upon his knowledge of anatomy and physiology and developed in the belief that science could be applied beneficially to physical education. In Czechoslovakia the Sokol movement was different again. Founded in 1862 by Dr Miroslav Tyrs the name Sokol means falcon, a bird of legendary courage, and a symbol of the nation's determination to remain independent. Sokol believed his exercises enabled individuals to take control of their own life and future. The Movement became well known for holding mass displays of physical training, but they were significantly different from those taking place in Germany. The Sokol system was purely voluntary and was established as a free democratic organisation. A major Sokol Festival was held in Prague in 1948 with guests from the UK, America, Russia, France, Belgium, Poland and the Scandinavian countries, as a celebration of their survival after the occupation during the war.

In Germany and Italy however, fitness training was beginning to be used for military ends. By 1936 the Nazi regime was in control and Hitler had started a rearmament process and his policies and mass rallies with his emphasis on compulsory fitness were viewed with considerable suspicion in Britain. It needs to be remembered that it was the nature of the rallies rather than the exercises themselves that were discredited. Some of the exercise movements in Germany, such as that of Rudolf Laban, predated the Nazis. He developed a form of dance with an emphasis on free expression, in marked contrast to the State's focus on regimentation. Others, like Heinrich Medau, followed Laban and developed forms of exercise that were based on dance, and were performed to music.

THE IDEAL

The vision of Mary Bagot Stack was for a world of peace and love. As she wrote herself:
'Human Health and Beauty are but stepping stones to that ideal'.

Her concept of 'beauty' was, like Keats, that 'Beauty is truth – Truth, Beauty'. She believed that a person's health and fitness were their own responsibility but that everyone should have the opportunity to take control of this aspect of their lives. To provide the means for them to do this became Mary's dream. It is clear that the horrors of the First World War had a deep impact on her. As an idealist, she had a romantic vision of how the world could be, as she wrote:

'Peace must finally come to this world by our own determination to make it come. Each individual can plant a weed or a flower in "Life's Garden". It is my belief that the health training and happy social contacts which we members find in our League are going to help us in our little corner of this vast universe to grow a few humble flowers.'

Mary's ideals were far reaching but she was realistic enough to know that she needed to be practical and take each step as it came. Each stage of the development of the League took faith and courage, and there is no doubt that her personal confidence and conviction helped to ensure the support of others and the League's ultimate success. In the last 75 years society has changed greatly in its attitudes to exercise and the role of women, and yet the League continues to be as relevant today as it ever was. The secret of a successful organisation: motivated leaders, open mindedness, adaptability and a willingness to continue to learn, have been at the heart of the League's success. This has not all been easily achieved, as unavoidable differences and debates have been a part of the process. The ultimate unifying force has been the strength of the central ideal which has remained at the heart of the League. Whether Mary could have envisaged that the worldwide organisation she created, would still be thriving seventy five years later, it is not possible to say. It would surely be a source of great satisfaction for her, even if world peace remains just a dream.

FAMILY AND FRIENDS

Prunella Stack was just twenty when her mother died and she not only took on full responsibility for the League but for fulfilling her mother's dreams. Her aunt Norah was there to help, taking on much of the administrative responsibility. The full and fascinating stories of Mary, her sisters and daughter can be found in books written by Prunella, 'Movement is Life' (1973) and 'Zest for Life and the League of Health and Beauty' (1988).

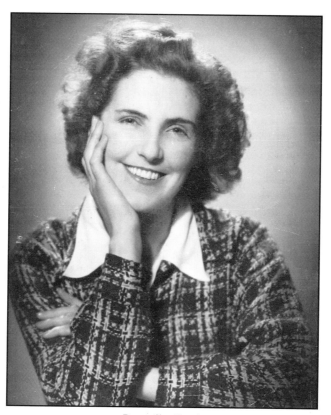

Prunella Stack

Prunella has been central to the League's success and survival. Whilst not always being personally at the helm because of family and other commitments, she has remained the predominant inspiration. She inherited her mother's charm and charisma, both being adroit at public speaking and able to win over audiences of any size. She has also performed a significant public role on various national bodies relating to health and exercise, and so in an indirect way the influence of the League has permeated many subsequent social developments.

Interwoven into the story of the League are the stories of many remarkable women who, like Prunella, have worked hard to ensure Mary's legacy was not lost. Peggy and Joan St Lo, two of Prunella's childhood friends, were paramount in the life of the League from the late 1930's. Their skills and knowledge combined to enrich the work of the League and ensure the high standards that Mary established. Many more were pioneers in different ways, with newly trained teachers taking the League to Centres all over the UK and even other countries, whilst others created the essential music that complemented the movement and exercise in classes and public displays.

THE BOOK

Each chapter has a central theme and although the sequence is guided by chronology, the middle chapters focus on the essential elements of the League's work, the Displays, the music, the magazine, the Second World War and the development of the League overseas. To tie events together there is an Appendix which lists all the key events in the League's history. A second Appendix explains, to those not familiar, the basis of the League's exercise system.

It is appropriate on the 75th anniversary to celebrate the League's success by looking back and recording the memories and experiences of the leaders, trainers and members, over the decades, to help us gain an insight into the heart and soul of the League.

"The finer the dream, the greater the thrill of even partial realisation", Mary Bagot Stack.

CHAPTER 2

THE DREAM

MARY BAGOT STACK

Many of us have dreams but how many of us know how to make them a reality? To understand the League, we need to look back on the life of its founder, Mary Bagot Stack. Her idealism and profound belief in the importance of movement, exercise and dance for the physical and spiritual well being of women, inspired her to build her dreams into a reality.

Mary Bagot was born in Dublin on the 12th June 1883, and amongst her family she was called 'Mollie'. Her sister, Norah wrote about her as a lively and good tempered child. When only eight years of age she developed peritonitis, and in those days, little could be done and she was very lucky to have survived. When she was fourteen, her father, who had invested all his money in the founding of the Dental Hospital in Dublin, was stricken with paralysis. A much heavier burden of responsibilities around the home fell to Mary, as the oldest of the three remaining children. Her three older siblings had already left home, among them, her older sister Nan who was studying in Paris. As Norah put it:

> 'Mollie gave up her work and became our father's right hand, our mother's steadfast help and comfort. I suppose some girls might have taken this necessity amiss. We had all been brought up to regard self-support not only as incumbent on us, but as a source of happiness, indeed, our passion was for independence. Mollie felt as strongly as the rest of us. She had no desire to settle down and be the daughter to stay at home. But she never complained, just continued to be her old cheery self, giving always all she had to all of us. We used to have marvellous parties in those days, always organised by her. We had no money at all and our drawing room was only about fourteen feet square, but we managed to give dances there, sitting out on the stairs.'

When Mary was seventeen she developed rheumatic fever which left her unable to pursue her studies and meant any ideas of a future career or independence seemed lost. Her illness did not diminish her determination to lead an independent life and this led her to seek out a form of exercise that would improve her health and well being.

EARLY INFLUENCES

Mary first met Mrs Josef Conn in 1906 whilst on a visit to see Nan, in Paris. Nan was eager to encourage Mary to find an interest outside her duties at home and took her to Mrs Conn's Institute. Mary had not experienced good health since her bout of rheumatic fever, and was interested in following up all new approaches to exercise. Mrs Conn taught remedial exercises, which had been specifically designed for women. Her classes included those who had been referred by doctors for treatment, as well as members of the general public.

Mrs Conn had learned many of her exercises from Sir Frederick McCoy, a doctor and professor at Melbourne University, and he in turn had been influenced by his knowledge of gynaecology and the physical poise and balance techniques used by the Ancient Greeks. The principles of the exercise systems developed by Conn and subsequently, Mary Bagot Stack can also be traced back to the Swedish system of gymnastics devised by Ling. In 1907 Mrs Conn opened a new Institute in London. Mary made her first break with home, when in 1908 she went to London to study under Mrs Conn. Her plan was to train as a teacher of exercise and then to return home and give classes in Dublin. Mary began to see improvements in her own health after a relatively short time, and she observed similar improvements in the fitness of the referred patients. The results were so positive that Mary changed her plans and decided to learn more. Mary worked hard and qualified in six months, and was invited to join Mrs Conn's staff.

The upsurge of interest in physical education and dance in Britain was predominantly amongst women. There were several women who had developed physical training courses in colleges, and dancers who were exploring wider forms of dance and movement. Mary Bagot Stack differed from most in that she devised her own forms of exercise outside of the education system and incorporated exercise, dance and movement into one form. As Margaret Peggie explained, it was the more traditional and formal aspects of Ling's exercises that were to be the main influence on the development of physical education in Britain, with the first Physical Education college opening in 1885. The number of colleges increased and were managed by women for women. Similarly in the world of dance, new ideas and new forms were emerging, much of it inspired by Isadora Duncan. Some of the leading exponents of modern dance in Britain were Margaret Morris, Madge Atkinson and Ruby Ginner. Ginner called her new dance form Revived Greek dance, and Mary was familiar with all of these.

The importance of these developments was that they offered women new opportunities for physical freedom, and to be able to extend their lives outside of family and work, and even for some into a career. Within this ongoing cultural context, Mary created her own unique style and approach, in relation to the exercises she developed. More significantly she was the first person to offer this experience to all women regardless of age or social class and this was in marked contrast to the courses offered by the women's colleges. Whilst these continued with more formal exercise regimes, Mary emphasised the role of relaxation, and rhythmic movements set to music.

HAPPINESS AND GRIEF

In the summer of 1909, whilst on a visit back home to Dublin, Mary met Captain Hugh Bagot Stack of the 2nd Battalion 8th Gurkhas who was home on leave from India. They had met years before but this latest meeting was different, their feelings for each other had grown, and before Hugh's leave was over, they were engaged. It was not possible for them to be married immediately, so Hugh returned to India and Mary to London. That autumn, Mary and Nan took their mother on her first break since their father's illness. Unfortunately while they were away, he died quite suddenly. This marked the end of family life in Dublin.

Mary took her mother with her when she went to Yarmouth to begin her teaching career, and later they moved to Manchester. Mary worked hard and was very successful and by the end of 1911 the marriage was planned. Hugh came home on leave in 1912 and they were married in the March, in London. After a long holiday in Ireland, Mary and Hugh set sail for India. In letters home she expressed her happiness and she was soon fully involved in the life of the Regiment.

Her interest in physical exercise and movement led her to wish to learn more about yoga. She found herself a teacher, a Mr Gopal, who tutored her in Hindu philosophy and yoga. He sent a yoga teacher to Mary's home to instruct her in the yogic asanas (the positions central to yoga) and relaxation techniques. She also became fascinated by the natural grace of the Indian women. She observed that this was due to the looseness and freedom of their movements and the adherence to habits of posture that no longer existed in Western countries. Mary began to see the possibilities for combining remedial exercises, yoga movements and posture training.

When in 1913 Mary became pregnant, Nan was very worried about her staying in India. News was received that Mary had had a son, and had called him Peter, but this news was soon marred by the baby's death at only two days old. Although her sorrow was great, she knew that she wanted another child and she became pregnant again soon after. On the day that Prunella was born, July 28th 1914, war was declared between Austria and Serbia. Two weeks later Hugh sailed for France. Mary knew that she had to return to England. Mary and Prunella set sail from India at the beginning of October, but with the slowness of transport, did not arrive back in England until November. In the meantime a telegram had been delivered to the family telling them that Hugh had been killed within a week of arriving in France. They did not know if Mary had been told, but she had discovered the terrible news as she arrived in England, from the Casualty Lists in the newspapers. The rest of the family then decided to make their home there as well to be a support for each other and Mary, and a home was established in London. At that point in her life when all must have seemed so desolate, alone with a small baby, she now had her loving family around her.

A NEW START

Mary stayed in London throughout the war sharing a flat with her sisters, looking after Prunella, and working each Sunday in a munitions factory. When peace came she wanted to do something practical to help other women, as she had seen the poor conditions in which most of them worked. Mary, with her interest in exercise and posture, was able to appreciate what benefits a wide range of different approaches to fitness and health could offer. To the many influences Mary had already experienced were added the Greek dance style of Ruby Ginner. However, Mary had her own ideas. She believed that the Conn system did not have sufficient emphasis on relaxation, and flowing movements, and so she created exercises, for fitness and posture incorporated with movement to music. She believed that the music not only added an element of enjoyment to the exercise routine but she also recognised the role of rhythm in guiding body movement.

Mary began to offer classes in exercise and dance for both women and children.

She began with children's exercise classes in her drawing room once a week, initially just for Prunella, her cousin Cinderella and their two friends Peggy and Joan St Lo, who Mary nicknamed 'Nobella' and 'Umbrella'. Their close friendship was to last the rest of their lives. This impromptu class became the starting point for larger children's classes at the Mayfair Hotel, and evening classes for business girls, at her home. These classes included many different forms of dance which aimed to teach people to move in the right and natural way using music as the means whereby this could best be achieved. With practice, the aim was to make the rhythm 'ripple through the whole body like a wave', and in time help the student to be responsive to more subtle rhythms. At the same time she was treating patients sent to her by doctors, some with asthma, and others with bone disorders.

From the outset the emphasis for Mary Bagot Stack was on movement rather than pure dance or exercise. There are many differences and similarities between these three forms, and as Margaret Peggie explains, 'movement' can be defined as 'somewhere between exercise and dance':

> ' 'Exercise' refers to that human physical activity which, in that it is designed to improve the physique and promote health and fitness, is therapeutic or remedial in intention. The term 'movement' refers to that kind of human physical activity where the emphasis is on exploring the variety of movement possibilities which the body is capable of, to improve the physical range and strength of the body. 'Dance' is even more problematic to define: it is a means of producing movement to a consideration of its possibilities as an art form.'

By 1923 Mary felt ready to give lectures and demonstrations and hired the Aeolian Hall. She approached the King's physician Lord Dawson of Penn and asked him to chair her meeting, and he agreed! This brought her more pupils and a chance to write articles for the press. As Mary's classes became increasingly popular she opened a training school to train others to be teachers of her methods. Further expansion did not seem possible with the complete lack of funds. With help from Nan, two years later in 1925, a larger house with a studio was bought in Holland Park. Nan converted the top rooms for letting and Mary began to recruit students.

SUCCESS

Mary Bagot Stack opened her Health School in 1925 at the house in Holland Park. In 1926 she recruited Marjorie Duncombe who had been recommended to her by Ruby Ginner, to help her with the teaching. Marjorie had trained as a dancer from a very early age. She had graduated from a three year course with Ginner in 1923 at the age of nineteen, and went on to Teacher Training College. Whilst maintaining her own classes, Marjorie also taught at Mary's School. She taught Greek dancing, ballet, national dancing, mime and voice production while Mary taught health exercises, ballroom dancing and public speaking. Together they put on displays that combined health and dance movements, with Mary also lecturing on health and exercise.

The first ten students on the two year course, included Joan and Peggy St Lo.

Peggy had begun her physical training seriously at the age of fourteen, and was a very gifted dancer, always the envy of others. Joan was two years older than Peggy, and she worked alongside her sister in all that they did. More than anything else Mary was impressed by Joan's constant good humour and welcomed her ability to make others laugh. Prunella trained between 1927 and 1930 and graduated when she was just sixteen, and after a year away at boarding school, she began to teach for the League at the age of seventeen.

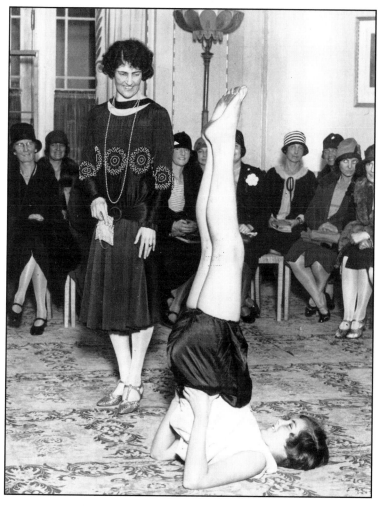

Mary Bagot Stack with Prunella 1926

When the first students graduated, all but Joan and Peggy became teachers. On completing the course, two years later, Prunella continued to work closely with her mother, whilst Peggy and Joan developed their careers on the stage. Joan was the first to get a professional booking and appeared in the chorus of the stage production of 'Lucky Girl' at the London Pavilion. She was joined shortly afterwards by Peggy whose chance came when another dancer left. Peggy's skills as a teacher were soon recognised and at the age of just seventeen, she was asked to become the ballet mistress to the chorus. In the mean time the two sisters lost no opportunity to learn many new dances, including tap. After eighteen months, the show was due to travel to America, but Joan and Peggy decided not to go with them. The sisters returned to Mary's school and began to teach. They brought with them their experience of the discipline of dance and the skills of choreography, which were to become the basis of the class work and central to many displays. Peggy's perfectionism and Joan's natural good humour, represented what were to become two of the main foundations of the League, high standards and a sense of fun.

THE DREAM

Never one to sit back and feel satisfied with her achievements, Mary had visions of a better world, where there was peace not war, and people were healthy and happy. Memories of the horrors of the First World War and ominous signs of ongoing troubles in Europe, with another war an increasing possibility, served to focus her mind in this direction. She believed strongly in 'the glory of unselfish giving' and in health and fitness for all. Mary taught her daughter Prunella that the more luck and good fortune she had, the greater her duties and responsibilities. Mary's sister Nan was no less visionary. She was convinced that leisure would be the 'problem' of the twentieth century. Soon there would be so much time that people would not know what to do with it as machines took over their work.

Mary held on to this dream of a different future not just for herself but for all women, the society in which she lived and for the world. By the late 1920's Mary was holding an evening class once a week for women who worked in London offices and shops. She had realised that teaching in these classes was a very different experience from working with the students at the Conn Institute. She wanted to extend her work to the women who she felt needed it most, office, shop, factory and mill workers and for children from poorer districts. Mary noticed the improvement in the physique of her pupils, and she wanted to provide more classes for all women at a price that they could afford. She looked to the Sokol movement in Czechoslovakia which aimed to unite youth through 'service through the medium of perfect self development', and thought that a similar organisation could be established for women, in the UK.

Mary later wrote about this time and how she had become inspired to begin the League:
　　'How do you get ideas? I get mine in my bath!'

To gain an appreciation of her enthusiasm, it is worth reproducing her account in full, as her personality shines through in her expressive writing style.

　　'According to my grandiloquent hopes we women were to start to build 'A new World', a world of Health, of Peace, of Happiness. Where to begin? What to begin? How to begin? Have you dear reader ever felt completely flummoxed – ever been faced with a blank and high mental stone wall? If you have – SHAKE!

　　I'll tell you what I did. I set my hard faced friend – my alarm clock – to 6.45 a.m. When it rang with that slap on the brain which sends all day and night dreams flying, I jumped out of bed, said my prayers had a cold bath, opened my windows, stripped off my clothes and set going on my gramophone the gayest jazz tune I could find, and I exercised around my bedroom, in physical bliss but mental blankness.

Suddenly in the middle of these bodily activities, I found I was thinking – thinking hard. My brain (such as it was and unfortunately still is) was beginning to work. Ideas came and came and more ideas came until at last they were pouring in so fast I could not catch them. Some mental tap had been unloosed from somewhere – from where, who knows?

Mental inertia was going, mental alertness was coming. I opened my windows wider, I breathed deeper, I leaped higher – mentally and physically I was bathed in gladness. Laziness – mental and physical – (the root of most failure) was going – and then – the BIG IDEA came. If energy is the source of life, and if we women want – as we all do Life, WE MUST HAVE ENERGY.

How? A league – A League of Women who will renew their energy in themselves day by day. A league of women pledged (so as to keep us lazy things at it) TO BREATHE TO LEAP - and, above all, to THINK.

A league with an on=my=honour=split =in=the=midriff promise in it. What fun! Oh, what fun!

Furiously I picked up a pencil and made notes of HOW TO BEGIN – HOW TO GO ON – HOW TO GO ONNER. (If dear reader, you are just now horrified at my illiterate style, forgive me – I can feel this very minute the tumbling excitement, the fury, the fun of the FIRST GREAT PUSH, i.e. getting the League down on paper – I did not then foresee the misery of getting it off the paper again. The anxieties, the crowding responsibilities, the indecisions and decisions. Those came later.)

I only saw before my eyes, in letters of flame, "THE WOMEN'S LEAGUE." League of what? League of Energy? No that would be too terrifying to the lazy, a frontal attack, always dangerous. League of Health? Our aim was going to be Racial Health. But no, that was utterly dull; it had none of that sparkle most women love – sparkling necklaces, bangles, rings, and eyes – sparkling thoughts, too, surely! League of ? – League of? – Oh dear! oh dear! Oh dear... Then floated into my mind – "build-the-body-beautiful" – the title of the book that I had just begun to write. A Build The Body Beautiful League?

I see now how unsuitable was the title. But the big "B" for Beauty – the ideal Beauty which I was writing about in my book attracted me, and so eventually our first endeavours started under that clumsy title.'

It is important to note that Mary's use of the term 'racial health' meant health for ALL inhabitants of the country and the world. Racial equality was a principle she held dear. As she wrote later:

'We have a very high ideal in the League. But then, if you don't hitch your wagon to a lofty star, how can you ever lift yourself above the rut of everyday life and routine? And so our idea is RACIAL HEALTH. Think of it for a minute! The complete absence of world disease from our modern vocabulary! Each life lived to its utmost, because there is no hampering ill-health to hold back its fulfilment! All those secret hopes and longings, which each of us stores in our hearts, made realities because the body is a glorious asset, instead of a handicap in the race of life.'

Mary decided that she must act on her new idea and she continued to describe her later thoughts and feelings.

'My heart sang all day to the lilt of the three B's – Build – Body – Beautiful. And at night, sleepily, I muttered "Build the Body Beautiful" – beautiful – what is Beauty? In a hazy, very indefinite way, the definition of which I have since made use came to me – "the thrill of worthwhile achievement" – that would be beautiful.

You see in my sleepy mind there were already in our League millions of members: our aim – racial health – was already achieved; peace and happiness were world wide! So, sleepily, I felt – VERY BEAUTIFUL!

In the middle of the night I awoke with a start from a financial nightmare. Warfare was afoot, a very subtle form of warfare. The belligerents were Rent v. Racial health. In the dark I lay and thought anxiously. If I dropped my private school and went into the arena of life to form a huge League, how could it be financed?

The source of my finances lay chiefly in my school: my daughter had to be educated – my rents had to be paid – my-my-my – I-I-I – I was already forging my own chains, putting the brake on my own endeavour.

Then my thoughts grew hazy, my anxious head cuddled down on the pillow, my dreams came back – Beauty – The Thrill Of Worth While Achievement… And in the night, believe me or not as you choose – I heard a voice saying, "Back the League."'

Many of us have dreams. But do we also have the faith to act on them? Following a dream is treading a new path and not knowing where it will take us. There has to be a large measure of serendipity as well as focused effort, but most of all there has to be a belief in what we want to achieve. This belief never left Mary.

CHAPTER 3

THE REALISATION

THE DREAM MADE REAL

The Women's League of Health and Beauty was a dream made real by Mary Bagot Stack's hard work and strong faith. Very few around her knew of her illness. That she was publicly praised for her health and vitality merely adds to the stature of her achievements.

The League began in March 1930 at YMCA premises in Regent St. There were a number of fully trained teachers already available from the ex-students of the Bagot Stack Health School. Among the sixteen foundation members were: Marjorie Morris, Violet Head, Lillie White, Edna Pritchard, Edith Ormsby-Taylor and Mary Preston. This gave the League its first capital of £8. One teacher, Doris Stark, writing later, recalls the first night:

> 'An excited Mrs Stack looked lovely. I can see the scene now - the cherry-coloured curtains and window seats all around the hall on which she periodically stood to get an all-round view of her class. The colossal ledgers she came armed with – a record was to be kept of the girls' weekly attendance – she said we must be methodical. But, of course, the idea had to be abandoned after the first couple of nights as the numbers were too great.'

Mary laid out her founding principles, which in fact became the principles which the League has followed ever since: self funding; large numbers and cheap prices so no-one was excluded, and expert instruction. The venture had begun without any sponsorship or financial capital, relying totally on the hope that as long as enough members joined it could be self supporting. The success of the first few months of the League was very encouraging for Mary. She decided that she should hire a large hall in central London to which she transferred her evening classes, which were soon attracting seventy or eighty women per session. To ensure most women could afford to attend, the classes cost only sixpence with a membership subscription of two shillings and sixpence.

Prunella remembers these times for her mother as being ones of constant work, with a very heavy, albeit, self imposed, schedule. Mary was effectively working three shifts, daytime, evening, and night. Daytime was her teaching and administrative work at the school, evening was when she taught League classes and the night time was when she planned the League's development. This was a schedule that would put a strain on even the healthiest among us. Three months after the League had begun, without making any fuss or complaint, Mary had undergone an operation to remove an enlarged thyroid gland in her neck. Unfortunately the thyroid gland had 'burst' and it was not possible to remove the whole of the enlargement. Her doctors told her that if the swelling were to return then this would be a serious set back. Undaunted she returned to work.

SPREADING THE WORD

Over the first months the League was succeeding in meeting its financial commitments from its income, due to the rapidly increasing membership. This was just the beginning, and Mary realised that it would take continuing effort and enterprise to ensure the League's growth and survival. This immediate success had proved to Mary that once women discovered the classes, they were enthusiastic and keen to tell others, however word of mouth alone would not be sufficient, Mary wanted women everywhere to have the chance to join. As is typical of her intuitive and original thinking she found an inspirational way to let the British public know of her new organisation and her ideals. As Margaret Peggie wrote:

> 'In her efforts to recruit new members, she revealed a remarkable flair for creating publicity ....In the beginning, knowing she could not pay for extensive advertising and with her customary audacity, she organised a public display in Hyde Park which attracted widespread interest from the press as well as from women who wanted to become members. Within six moths there were over a thousand members in the London area.'

This foundation demonstration was held on the 12th June in the Cockpit, Hyde Park. There were many comments in the press after this event:

> 'The League of Health and Beauty (was) founded to give London women health classes at sixpence each lesson. In Germany, Sweden and Switzerland where the science of health is a progressive and national responsibility, similar physical culture demonstrations are events of public importance.'

Such positive publicity helped considerably in getting the crowds to the display and increasing membership.

Word was spreading beyond the capital, and it soon became clear that there was a need to open centres elsewhere. By the end of the first year the membership in London had risen to over two thousand and there was no longer sufficient room in the hired halls. Mary knew that she needed a large, permanent premises but wondered how she was to achieve this with just £180? One venue which she knew would be ideal was the Mortimer Halls in Great Portland St, in the West End of London but that would cost £2,000 per year in rent. Rather than settle for less she began to work out a way to raise the necessary funds. Mary did not ask others for help and focused instead on introducing additional classes, and recruiting new members. Mary was not going to wait for circumstance to help her, she, as always, gave it a hefty push. She wrote a letter to all members asking them to increase their attendances and to bring in new members. This was a pure act of faith on her part and took a great deal of courage. She signed the lease, using her private resources and life insurance as a guarantee against the rent.

A report in the League magazine by League pianist Deidre Welsh, describes the move to Mortimer Halls:

> 'Then came the chaos of those early days at Mortimer Halls which gradually resolved into the orderly timetable of a great headquarters of a

famous movement, with snack bar, four halls with continuous classes every evening, a hive of offices, and eighty to a hundred students training in the daytime to become teachers. I remember too the afternoon classes at the Mayfair hotel, taken by Mrs Stack personally.'

There was no time for Mary to relax. But by January 1931 the swelling had returned in her neck and she once again consulted her specialist. She was told that unless she underwent an immediate operation with no guarantee of permanent recovery, she would live for only six or eight months, probably much less, but even with an operation chances were small of a permanent recovery. Mary had just signed the lease of Mortimer Halls and had innumerable responsibilities. She knew that it was too soon for her to give up all she had worked for. As Prunella recollects she believed that if she stopped, the League would not survive. She decided not to have the operation. Mary reasoned that the doctors might be wrong and she wanted to rely on the power of prayer and a belief that the body was its own best doctor. She was convinced that she would be spared long enough to establish the League on a sound permanent basis. She wrote at the time:

'What shall happen to our League matters more to me than life itself'.

Her vitality and faith were so strong that those around her found it difficult to believe that she was so ill. The time left to her also gave her the opportunity to groom her daughter Prunella to take over her work.

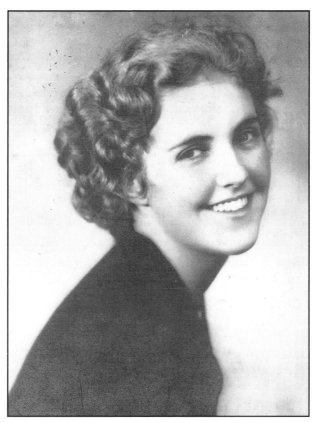

Prunella Stack 1930

THE WIDER CONTEXT

By 1930 although subtle changes were occurring in society in relation to what was an acceptable role for women, and physical training colleges had become established, there was little official interest in exercise, and those in positions of power in the colleges and on government bodies, had a vested interest in maintaining the status quo. So it was that the League's work developed rapidly without any official blessing. However, such was the success of the League and its mass appeal to women that it began to be noticed by those in positions of influence. There was also the beginnings of awareness at Government level of movements in Europe which focused on producing a healthy population, whether this was envisaged to be as a workforce or a military force. In a new venture, the Board of Education supported exercise classes in schools which were financed by local education authorities and other forms of keep fit began to emerge. Government sponsored schemes were set up alongside the work of Mary Bagot Stack, and followed a different type of exercise regime.

Although the teachers of keep fit usually came from Women's Colleges of Physical Training, some of those in charge of the colleges were vocal opponents of Mary Bagot Stack's work and the League. Dr Anna Broman, a doctor and a physical educationalist was very strong in her disapproval; she felt that there was a need for educationally trained gymnasts to be the only ones who should be allowed to take classes. She wished to stop 'this reckless and uneducated enthusiasm' for the League, and thus to protect her own position of influence over the Physical Training Colleges and the newly emerging keep fit movement. The overwhelming success of the League was a very real threat to this. History shows that tides can only be held at bay or redirected for a limited time, and change was inevitable. None of the wider developments in keep fit interrupted the continuing growth of the League, or could challenge its popularity. What the 'educationalists' chose to ignore was the lengthy and extensive training that League teachers underwent with a full time course over two years which covered anatomy, physiology and kinesiology, as well as specific exercise and dance classes. This enhanced the credibility and confidence of all involved.

MEMBERSHIP SOARS

Mary continued to work hard and the growth of the League continued apace. The first suburban Centre was soon opened at Golder's Green. The pianist for the event, Deidre Welsh, wrote of Mrs Stack's 'amazing vitality and personality'. So it was that despite her very poor health Mary continued to inspire others and at the same time she seemed to gain in strength from her deeply held ideals. In a speech in 1932 she said:

> 'Why have we called our League a League of Health and Beauty? Because we want eventually to travel far beyond the region of just health; that is only a first step. When I speak of beauty I never mean just physical beauty – beauty of the arched eyebrow, the chiselled nose, the short upper lip – but the beauty that shows in its outer radiance and inner harmony of body and spirit. This beauty is worth achieving, and yet the more one thinks of beauty, the more one realises it is such a far goal that it will probably mostly remain on the top of the mountain peak wrapt in

mystery, disclosing itself only in rare moments. Perhaps, indeed, beauty is something one feels, rather than something one sees.'

In 1931 membership was five thousand but by 1932 it stood at twenty thousand. During that year many more Centres opened including Liverpool which was the third Centre opened by Mary Bagot Stack, and the first one in Scotland, in Glasgow. In that year, it was also decided to introduce a League uniform. This was for the members to wear whilst exercising, and was intended to level out any differences in age and social background, that might be exhibited by clothing. Exercise wear was not available in shops, so Mary's sister Nan designed black satin pants and a white satin blouse, to be worn by all members. Exposing so much bare leg was very daring for that time. The garment design was such that it should not impede movement and although the pants became shorter over the years, the style remained unchanged. Patterns for members to make their own outfits were available as well as the ready made items. Short skirts and small capes could be added if required and these were used for the marches.

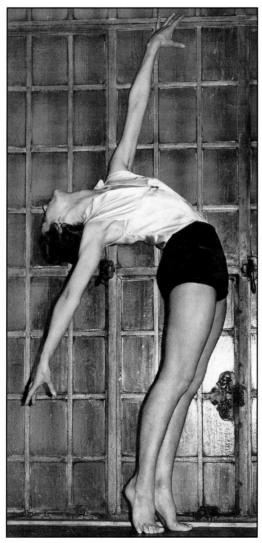

Peggy St Lo in League Uniform

The visit to Hyde Park in the summer was already becoming a tradition, with the third display to be held there and the second show at the Albert Hall. Hundreds of women in mini black velvet skirts and capes walked down Oxford Street shepherded by policemen for whom such public gatherings were unfamiliar. This was also a new sight for passers by, seeing so many women 'swinging' along behind a military band! At the Albert Hall Mary Bagot Stack announced that the League was planning to produce a magazine, which was to be called 'Mother and Daughter'. She said that its aim was 'to find only the best and the beauty in all.'

This was also the first year that the League held beach classes at Bournemouth. These attracted the attention of the Star newspaper, which decided to organise tours with a selected team of teachers to visit a different town every three days for three weeks during the summer. The Star then arranged an evening out at a London show and a dinner at the Savoy for the team at the conclusion of the tour. The publicity and general approval of the League and its work was still very strong in the media.

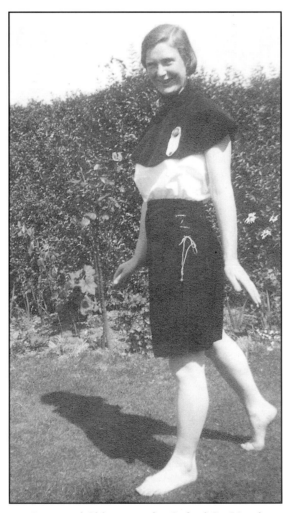

Cape and Skirt worn for Oxford St. March

By 1933 the membership had grown to over thirty thousand in Great Britain alone. The audience for the Hyde Park demonstration was a record thirty thousand, and with many more participants the evening display was again at the Albert Hall. Men's trial classes were held that year, the outcome of requests from members for the League to organise something for brothers, husbands and sons. A qualified male instructor was found and the exercises were done to music. It was decided that the men attending these classes would not be required to be enrolled as members, and that they would continue as long as there was a demand. No further reference to this experiment could be found! Fortunately, everything else set in motion that year was destined for success and longevity. There was the eagerly awaited publication of the first edition of 'Mother and Daughter', edited by A. J. Cruikshank, Mary's sister. The magazine had a silver cover and was produced quarterly.

By 1934 there were over forty seven thousand members and there were fifty students in training to be League teachers. The Daily Mirror asked Mary to write a series of articles for them on slimming, which she did. At this time the League was probably the only organisation to rival the Women's Institute in size and popularity. New centres continued to open, and as exercise became a more established part of the culture of the country, other organisations were beginning to emerge, for example, Norah Reed was pioneering what was to become the Keep Fit Association.

A CREATIVE FOCUS

Mary had many family and friends who shared her enthusiasm and faith in what she was doing. Prunella was always very close to her mother at this time as were her two close childhood friends Peggy and Joan St Lo. The contribution of the two sisters was crucial. Even a short experience of the stage had taught Joan and Peggy skills that they could bring to their teaching for the League. In particular their expertise at presentation, choreography and arranging exercises to music helped to build a firm foundation for all the displays held since, setting high standards for the future. They became renowned for the discipline that they expected from their students.

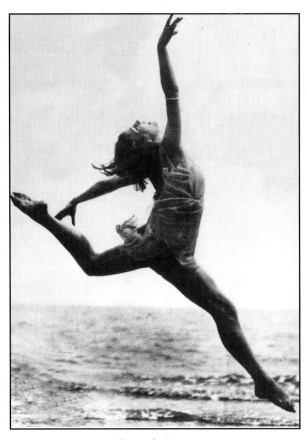

Peggy's Leap

It was a photo of Peggy that became the symbol of the League. Known as Peggy's Leap, it shows that from the tip of her toes to the angle of her head, there is a perfect radiation outwards, coming from a steady centre of control. This photo was taken on Clacton beach during a photo-shoot organised by the picture editor of the Times. The tide was out leaving a vast expanse of sand, which tempted Peggy and two companions to try a great leap. According to Prunella their back legs were supposed to be straight but Peggy's just lifted at the moment the photo was taken and the everlasting image was created. Mary could see that using the Leap as the League emblem epitomised grace and vitality, and was a true representation of its motto, 'Movement is Life'.

All the numbers choreographed by the St Lo sisters for performances, were added to the original sequences which had been created by Mary Bagot Stack, building up a formidable repertoire available to teachers. Peggy was the main producer of the Displays and Demonstrations. Her philosophy was that she should create items that were within the capability of the performers, and in that way she could ensure precision. In interview, League pianist Barbara Furniss, recollects:

> 'In the early days I worked with Peggy and Joan mainly. I was then a headquarters pianist. There were other teachers as well but Peggy and Joan ruled the roost. They were lovely people. All people were taught the Bagot-Stack way. Once they had the basics they could improvise. Peggy and Joan were wonderful at drawing out the best in people. They would encourage others to be creative. It was a great way to get people involved.

They had very great imaginations as they were always working to live music. We always had a march in, which we do not always do now. They would say 'Let's see some good walking'. It helped you get that feeling of poise.

Peggy and Joan were trained dancers. Their performance and their interest in movement and dance with the League, caught their imagination. They taught classes where every part of the body was explained, and every movement devised by Mrs Stack was for a specific part of the body. Using these movements Peggy and Joan did some wonderful sequences. They embodied the principles and they always had a theme. If it was an advanced waist movement then it was called 'Advanced Waist Movement'. So members and any audience knew exactly what they were looking at and where the concentration was needed. For displays there were prettier names.

Their attitude towards the League was quite phenomenal. They believed absolutely wholeheartedly in it. They knew exactly what they wanted from a performance, which they got. There was no messing about. They were very keen on teacher's training courses. They were devoted to the League. They sorted out a lot of the music themselves for the set items. Other than that, they were delighted if you provided something else for them.'

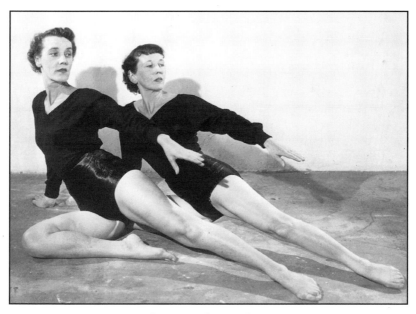

Peggy and Joan St Lo

By 1934 Peggy St Lo was the Head Teacher at the School and also involved in the administrative work. The compiling of the timetable was no small feat, given the rate at which the number of classes expanded. Joan partnered her in much of her work, and as Peggy was striving for technical perfection, Joan was more in touch with the performance. Joan could perform anything she was shown and had a good eye and memory for movement. It was up to her to remember what had been done and help Peggy put the sequences together. They were the perfect team.

MARY'S LEGACY

For the first four years of the League, Mary Bagot Stack had worked strenuously to promote and build the membership, travelling all over the country to support the efforts of all the Centres that were being established. Most who saw her remained completely unaware of her illness and that was how she wished it to be. She was frequently described as fit, healthy and beautiful, epitomising what the League stood for. Everything continued apace with the by now traditional rallies and displays. In May 1934 League members from all over the country assembled for a rally in London. It began with a service at All Soul's church, followed again by a march down Oxford Street and a display in Hyde Park, with a thousand members. The evening venue was held in front of a packed audience at the Albert Hall.

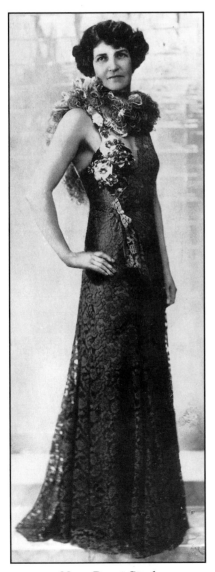

Mary Bagot Stack

However, by July 1934 Mary was seriously ill, with some doctors believing she had only weeks to live. She alternated between good and bad periods, but never gave up hope of recovery. This lasted for six months and she bore her illness with great courage. She died peacefully on January 26th 1935 aged just fifty one. The funeral took place at All Soul's church Langham Place on January 29th, and was attended by teachers and members from throughout the country. As the Minister giving the Address at her funeral said, the League was her memorial.

Prunella was well placed to continue her mother's work. Her life up to that point had been an excellent training ground, and her closeness to her mother and their shared strengths and beliefs, made her the ideal successor. She worked in the office by day, taught in the evenings and participated in the displays as both producer and performer. She had strong and loyal friends to help. After Mary's death Marjorie Duncombe gave up her other teaching and concentrated on her work with the League. Joan and Peggy thought that she was the League's best teacher, and following her methods, Peggy and Joan soon became the central focus for the training, displays and creative work of the League.

Post 1935, Prunella was also developing a role looking outside the League to see what was happening in the wider field of physical education and dance. She deemed it very important that the League stay abreast of developments and this involved her in taking trips to see for herself what was happening across Europe. In 1936 Prunella travelled to Germany and in Berlin she saw a number of physical systems of training, which included that of Rudolf Laban. The system she liked best was that of Heinrich Medau a colleague of Laban and in 1937 she spent a short time at his School of Gymnastics. From there she travelled to Czechoslovakia to see the Sokols who had inspired her mother. Upon her return to the UK, the travelling and public speaking continued, as many new centres opened across the country.

Prunella Stack was the idol of girls working in shops offices and factories in the 1930s, and had her early life and exploits written about in the newspapers of the day. This was an age without cynicism and Prunella's idealism and strengths, set her up as a role model. She was termed by the media: 'The Perfect Girl', and this was a great embarrassment to her.

RECOGNITION AND READJUSTMENT

In the face of the astounding success of the League, official acknowledgement had to follow. Organisations like the League with a focus on dance and movement, rather than just exercises, appealed to women rather than men and were far more popular than any other form of keep fit. Not everyone from the Physical Training Colleges disapproved of the League. Phyllis Colson recognised its value in extending physical training to the community at large. She later founded the Central College of Physical Recreation, which organised classes for teachers of 'keep fit' and in 1936 she established the Central Council of Recreative Physical Training. The Council had the support of the Board of Education and the Women's Colleges, and aimed to bring under its aegis all forms of sport, dance and physical training. The League was invited to become a member of the Council and its membership has been continuous ever since, except for during the war. The Council later changed its name to the Central Council of Physical Recreation. The shared purpose of Council members was to encourage more people into active participation in physical recreation, so that they might enjoy better health, as well as hopefully, having fun. Society was at last catching up with the thinking of Mary Bagot Stack!

The growth of exercise movements abroad and within Britain increased awareness of the benefits of developing a healthier populace, and in 1937 the British government created a Fitness Council with the remit to improve the health of the people of Britain. Prunella was invited to join this body in a letter from the then Prime Minister, Stanley Baldwin, which stated that 'Your knowledge and experience will, I am confident, prove of the greatest assistance to the Council.' As Prunella remarked,

> 'Of course I accepted! It was a flattering invitation for a twenty two year old and also a tribute to the League's standing.'

The idea that exercise should be for all, and be about movement rather than just exercises was also reinforced by the arrival in 1938 of Laban, a refugee from Nazi Germany. His approach influenced the training of keep fit and the provision of inexpensive classes for the general public. This was the first serious competition for the League. The work of Mary Bagot Stack was bearing fruit beyond the League.

The two great Displays in Wembley Stadium in 1937 and 1939 showed that nothing could dent the success of the League. The first was a Coronation Pageant to celebrate the crowning of King George VI, which had over five thousand members performing. The second in June 1939 had been planned as an International Festival but when Germany invaded Czechoslovakia, the political climate changed across Europe and the Display reverted to a more modest affair, but there were still over six thousand members participating. As Prunella wrote:

> 'Their performance on the green grass of Wembley's vast arena, lit by a mellow sun and later, as darkness fell, by dramatic spotlights, remained in the memory of many of the thousands who thronged the auditorium to watch them on that June evening in the last summer of peace.'

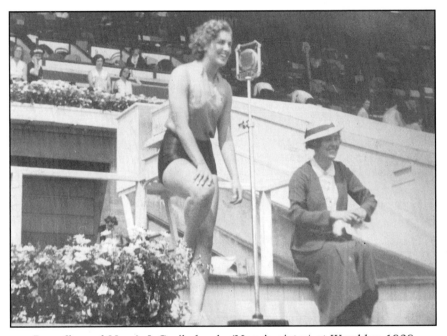

Prunella and Mrs A.J. Cruikshank. (Mary's sister) at Wembley 1939

The impending war with Germany had cast a shadow over the country but this was not allowed to interfere with life continuing as normal. In 1938 Prunella had married Lord David Douglas-Hamilton in Glasgow cathedral. This was a major social event in Scotland and for all her family and friends a special train was put on from London. This was also the year in which the first big rally was held in Scotland, at the University Athletics' ground in Glasgow. By 1939 the Daily Sketch had taken the League message to heart and regularly published news and pictures about the League, doing what they could to popularise their activities. However, it soon became clear that normal life was not destined to continue. The declaration of war brought the issue of survival rather than growth, to the fore. League membership stood at 166,000. The indomitable determination and hard work of Mary Bagot Stack and all her family and friends had given the League a solid foundation, which, with necessary readjustments, would ensure its survival.

War and peace were issues that had concerned Mary as early as 1932, when she wrote:

> 'What is likely to hinder us? – I suppose the two big human problems, disease of the body, and that disease of the international mind which we call war. Both of these should be classified under the one name Delay – and delay is dangerous. The law of life is Progress; if our League is to live it must sweep away delay and progress towards that next milestone where disputes have dispersed and harmony beckons. Peace will then be real and tangible instead of just a hope.'

CHAPTER 4

THE WAR AND ITS AFTERMATH

DISRUPTION

All aspects of social life were dramatically altered by the war and the League suffered badly. Women were needed in the workforce and many teachers had little choice but to stop running their classes and either enlist or do war work in industry. Those teachers remaining were helped in their efforts to maintain classes by members who were authorised as Practice Class Leaders. Together this small group continued as many classes as they could, in London and elsewhere, dodging air raids as they moved between venues. Across the country, new classes were also opened for office and factory workers, Civil Defence staff, Nurses and Service Personnel. In London fifty League Centres were kept open throughout the war. In the downstairs hall of Mortimer Halls, Peggy and Joan St Lo and Olga Roston continued taking classes, using the adjoining cloakroom as an office for the administration of the League. It was only during the 'Blitz' that the headquarters had to be closed. These combined efforts kept the League's work alive.

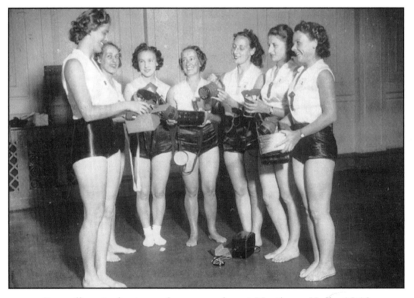

Prunella, students and gas masks at Mortimer Halls 1940

In London, one of the Centres that remained open was Surbiton and Sutton, and classes continued under increasingly difficult circumstances. For a short while, the loss of the local electricity station meant classes had to be held by candle light. Then when their hall was demolished by a bomb it was not possible to find another, so rather than give up their classes, members travelled to Thames Ditton each week. During the winter members went to classes armed with firewood and coal to try to heat their premises!

New centres continued to open despite all the problems. Among them was Belmont in Surrey, which opened in 1940, with one class for adults and another for children. These classes flourished and it was soon necessary to divide the children into three groups, babies, juniors and teenagers and to open an additional afternoon class for adults. Even though they spent more time in the air raid shelter than they did in the hall, the group never missed a single class and held extra Sunday morning classes to replace those that had to be abandoned.

There were other Centres which grouped together in their attempts to keep classes going, for example, those around Golders Green, Barnet, Hendon, and Finchley. When, owning to war work and evacuation, the classes in these areas dwindled or ceased the few members remaining continued their exercises at Joan Wilder's home in Hampstead Garden on Wednesday and Saturday afternoons. Joan, writing later, recalls:

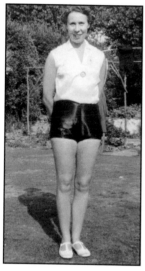

Joan Wilder

'For a while all went well. With a little furniture moving we were able to find room for about half a dozen people to work at the same time, blessing the efficient compactness of the League exercises. Then, at four in the morning of 16th November 1940, after more than six weeks' continuous nightly 'blitz', a blow, in the shape of a land mine a few yards from our front door, fell. From a cupboard beneath the stairs, I lay and watched bricks, glass and wood work hurled madly through the hall to settle like a macabre carpet, more than ankle deep. When the dust from falling ceilings cleared a bit and we had crawled out, shaken but uninjured, I surveyed the wreckage of the room through a gap torn in the crazily leaning wall, and from the stunned confusion of thoughts in my mind there rose to the surface the realisation that this was a Saturday and that there would be no classes that day, nor by the look of things, on any other.

Although there was fortunately no loss of life in this incident it caused widespread damage, and those members whom it had been impossible to warn arrived at their usual class time with rather white faces, having guessed at the situation of the explosion as they passed increasing evidence of it along their way from the bus stop. For some weeks while we were staying with friends various members generously offered the use of their homes for classes. In this way they were continued until the middle of December when we moved to another house.'

Not to be deterred by the destruction of her home, Joan continued classes, adding an extra evening class in 1941. On top of this she took League classes into factories and offices, and even the Civil Defence Service. She remembered:

'My recollections of this period consist mainly of long, dreary journeys in the cold and blackout, twice a week. More cheerfully I recall teaching through a microphone at Smith's clock factory in the canteen while the

Home Guard drilled in one corner and a First Aid class was held in another, with the clatter of washing up from behind. Every now and then a man pushing a huge trolley of rattling crockery proceeded slowly and solemnly through the lines of girls in my class.'

Joan's valiant attempts to continue League classes were curtailed when she was called up to work in the purchasing department of a factory. She then became aware of the effects on women of such sedentary work, and quickly devised some simple exercises that she could perform whilst sitting at her desk.

During the early years of the war members continued to rehearse for displays in aid of war charities, entertaining the wounded in hospital and supporting other local charities. This was made possible by teachers and members giving their spare time in the evenings. Around London, League items were organised for dances and cabarets in aid of Funds for the Forces, Wool funds, variety entertainments for members of HM Forces and Base Hospitals' Entertainment Committees, and socials for ARP and Ambulance Units and Wartime charities. A Revue held at King George's Hall, Great Russell Street, in London, raised funds for the Red Cross and St John's Ambulance Fund, while Salisbury members took part in a 'Wings for Victory' week.

Amazingly, the Summer Schools continued throughout the war, run by Peggy and Joan St Lo, and were based at the Manor House in Bookham. Anyone able to get leave joined the group and this was an opportunity for them to escape the war work for one short week, and to relax. Writing in the League magazine in 1992, Edith Strudwick recalled those days:

'During the War Practice Class Leaders had to attend a Summer School at Little Bookham where on fine days we would work in the lovely gardens pausing only when V.1s (flying bombs) approached and caused us to hide in the bushes! We slept in dormitories and when there was a night air-raid warning the martinet of a Housekeeper would rush round blowing a whistle and shouting 'Under your beds, girls.' From which we were only allowed to emerge when the all-clear went. I can still remember Joan and Peggy St Lo wearing their tin hats, gas masks at the ready, parading outside the buildings, taking their turns on fire-watching duties.'

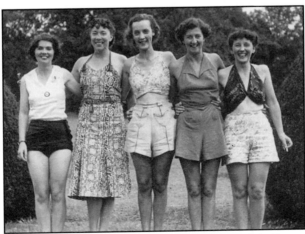

Little Bookham: l-r Marnel King, Deidre Welsh, Peggy St Lo, Kathleen O'Rourke, Joan St Lo.

Similar valiant efforts were occurring wherever there were League Centres. In Birmingham there were very few classes held in the evenings as most people would not go out at night during the blackout. Instead classes were held during the day and in the lunch hours of local firms. In both offices and factories new classes were established, such as the BSA factory and Lloyds House offices. These classes did not continue after the war, but many new members who had benefited from them stayed with the League.

In Scotland the Centres in Glasgow, Edinburgh, Ayr and Paisley remained open throughout the war. This was possible because advanced members who did their war work during the day, ran classes in the evenings. In 1940 Jean Yuill, who became a PTI sergeant during the war, managed to open a new centre in Lennoxtown. Her daughter Fiona Gillanders recollected her mother's stories from those years:

> 'People would walk miles to class in the dark and they could not carry lights. In Ayr the only pianist they could get was an old lady who played for the local church. All she could play was 'Yield not to Temptation' so she played that at different speeds!'

The magazine was not produced and there is scant record of what happened during the war years. The horrors of the war took their toll on League members and their families as they did on everyone. Among the many sad losses, in 1944 Prunella's husband who was in the RAF was killed, and she was left a widow with two small sons. Soon after when the war finally ended there was the huge task of getting life back to some semblance of normality. League members helped with parties around the country to celebrate the end of the war and the return of those in the armed forces. In 1945 at the London Thanksgiving week, the League's display in Trafalgar Square was one of the major attractions, seen by an audience of fifteen thousand.

RE-ESTABLISHING THE LEAGUE

The war was finally over, and although the League had continued in some areas, with changes of time and venues, there was a lot of work to be done to re-establish regular classes throughout the UK. How was this to occur? With sparse funds and no central full time organisers, what else but to rely on the spirit and resourcefulness of League teachers across the country. The ethos of resilience and determination had permeated those who had joined the League in the 1930's, clearly inspired by Mary Bagot Stack, Prunella, and Joan and Peggy St Lo. This was how the League had begun and it was how it would again prosper.

In 1946 the Bagot Stack Health School re-opened and by then thirty nine Centres had been re-established in London and in fifty three towns and cities across England and Scotland. In a Health and Beauty magazine article from early 1947, the activities of the League in 1946, the first year of peace, are described:

> 'On the one hand there was re-union, relief from strain, rehabilitation. On the other, queues, rationing, restrictions. Between these two extremes our lives continue, gradually becoming more normal, gradually adjusting themselves to the slow transition from war-time to peace-time conditions.

Once more, the planning and expansion of constructive work becomes possible. And in this field, the League has made the fullest use of its opportunities. Centres are re-opening. New members are joining. Results of the steadfast work of the keen members who 'carried on' during the war, are daily becoming more apparent.

Points of Progress. February – the re-opening of the Teacher's Training College. June – the League's first Peace-time rally and display at Wembley, where 1,500 members performed before an audience of 8,000 people. July – the League's team of 24 took part in the March Past at the large Festival of Youth staged by the Central Council for Physical Recreation (to which the League is now affiliated) at Wembley Stadium. July – seven teachers, who had taken the intensive six-months training, qualified and prepared to re-open Centres. August – the annual Summer School took place at Bognor Regis.

These are all concrete achievements, indicative of the League's vitality and the worth of its work. Constructive effort was never more needed in the world than it is today. The League, infused with its valuable spirit of happy comradeship, hopes it may play its part in re-building the life of the nation to the full.'

The focus of the earlier work was on London but this soon spread to the provinces, which is how the rest of England, was then referred to. Scotland, Eire, Northern Ireland Australia and Canada had all very quickly re-established Centres but the revival in Wales was still a few years away.

After the war a new trend emerged that has continued to this day. Members would join together to take weekend breaks and holidays. The summer break from classes did not mean a rest for all members as this became the time that many met to practice routines for local, area and national displays, but for most, when classes stopped for the summer, they wanted the opportunity to continue with their exercises and not just on their own. This is when a few individuals took the initiative and began booking holidays for League members from various Centres. Individual members saw this as an opportunity to meet members from other Centres as well as continuing exercising during the summer break. An early example of this is when Mary Bell booked a week at Duporth Holiday Camp in St Austell Bay on the Cornish coast. Members joined in from Stourbridge and Halesowen, Ilford, Reading and Southend. Exercise classes were held for an hour pre breakfast, leaving the rest of the day to tour or relax.

Efforts to recruit new teachers also began again. In 1947 Mary Lillis, met and was inspired by Kathleen O'Rourke, who soon convinced Mary to train as a teacher. As one of the first students to qualify in that year she described what it was like immediately after the war:

'I was, like all my generation, mentally and physically a victim of the times. I was one of the grey, drawn faces in the London Tube; too tired to rest; too restless to try.

There were seven of us on the course; seven who had known six years of war; six years of those things which deadened the mind and kill the spirit;

seven of us to awake one morning and feel that it was good to be alive: a possession not one of us had ever hoped to own again.'

It was this reawakened spirit of the newly trained teachers that over the next decade was to slowly ensure that the League once again spread to all the major towns. By the end of 1949 Centres had been re-established in most towns in England and the key cities in Scotland, Wales, Eire and Northern Ireland. Centres in Wales were not reopened until the early 1950's but other Centres had to wait even longer, like Oxford, which did not re-open until 1957.

BETTY'S MISSION

To understand what was involved in re-opening Centres, the experiences of Betty Urquhart illustrate well the determination, and belief that the teachers had in what they were doing. Betty had first joined the League in 1937 in Paisley, Scotland. Her first teacher was Seona Ross, shortly after followed by Jean Yuill, whom Betty describes as her inspiration. She attended classes regularly and so impressed Jean that she was asked to help with classes even though she was not yet trained. The war interrupted her plans to become a teacher but this was soon remedied when the war ended.

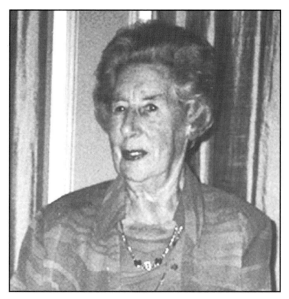

Betty Urquhart

When Betty had finished her teacher training in 1949, she did not return to Paisley but was asked to go to Cardiff to open all the Welsh Centres that had been closed during the war. In those days the League Executive Committee sent teachers where they were needed. At that time it was not expected that newly qualified teachers would return to their home groups, as it was felt that they might not have the necessary authority over women they had known all their lives. Aged twenty five, Betty was considered to be one of the older students, and she also had previous experience. Teachers, then as now, were self employed, but under special circumstances were subsidised by the League. Betty was given the sum of £48 to help her in the move. As Betty says:

'My mother thought I was mad, so did my older brother who was a bank manager. Well, one Saturday, I got on this train, and went to Cardiff... the confidence that you have at that age.... I wouldn't do it now. I thought, how on earth am I going to get started, I don't know anybody here! I got off the train at Cardiff and did not know a living soul. Well I managed to find this very third rate hotel but they only had a room for that night. Anyway the manager took pity on me and said I could keep my bags in reception and if I was to go back that evening, he would see if he had a free room. Well this went on for a few nights! On Monday morning I began my trek round Cardiff to get proper digs. Eventually I found digs with a Mrs Hughes. Finding digs wasn't easy, it being a university town. I had an attic room right at the top of the building, it was a four storey house, it was freezing cold with no heating.'

Betty lost no time in making contacts and trying to generate interest in the League. She planned to put on a big introductory evening, open to all, at the City Hall. First of all, though, she realised that she would need some help. She put an advertisement in the local paper asking if anyone who had once been a member of the League and who was interested in re-opening the classes, to meet her in the tea room at the Capitol cinema. One member turned up and willingly helped Betty for the next few weeks. For the opening night at the City Hall, Betty wanted to invite anyone who might be interested in the League, and others who she thought might have influence, so she included on the list the Medical Officer for Health. She also invited the nearest teacher, Joy Flanaghan, who lived in Weston super Mare, and Elizabeth Mallett who came down from London to do the official opening on behalf of the League.

'I managed to organise this opening which was absolutely wonderful, don't forget I was very naïve in all this, there were massive numbers of people there and they couldn't all join that night. The day before the opening, I had this brilliant idea. I went and hired a van with a loudspeaker, to tour the streets of Cardiff, thinking, that will bring them in! But what I did not realise was that I had a very broad Scots accent so no-one could possibly have understood what I was saying! So I do not know if people came out of sheer curiosity.

Anyway, so the opening was in September and we filled the Civic Hall, I remember I did a demonstration there with Joy. We did actually have some enrolments but not many. We started classes the next week at the High School. The classes are still at the High School. That first night I was with Kay a young teacher who was very raw, and she was going to do the reception for me. When we got to the High School, I remember saying to Kay, look there's a queue, there must be something else on at the school, as there was a new hall and an old hall and we were in the old hall. I had such a shock when I realised that the queue was all for us. It wound round the playground. We joined hundreds of members that night, and so we took off in Wales. One of my original members is still in Cardiff. That started me off, that was the Tuesday night, and then we opened an afternoon class. Then in about 1949 or 50 we moved on to Swansea and Newport and Penarth, so that was me full time.'

Betty is now eighty two and still runs six classes a week, across the West Midlands. Based in Droitwich Spa, she travels to Hagley, Birmingham, Stourbridge, Stourport and Wolverhampton. On top of this she runs an office in Droitwich which supplies leotards and other League clothing to members. It is remarkable women like Betty who have helped to make the League the organisation it is.

CHAPTER 5

THE LEAGUE MAGAZINE

EARLY EDITIONS

The first League magazine was produced in September 1933, and was entitled 'Mother and Daughter', with the aim: 'To find only the Best and the Beauty in all.' Mary Bagot Stack wanted the magazine to be a link between headquarters and the centres, and to be the mouthpiece through which she could talk to members. It was also hoped that it would result in 'large profits' which could contribute to the League's development. For the first few months Mary managed the magazine, press and publicity single handed. She soon realised that this was too much for her on top of the increasing demands on her as leader and teacher, so she invited her sister Mrs A. J. Cruickshank to become the editor. Mrs Cruickshank was the perfect choice as she was experienced in public relations and was already a regular contributor to various women's journals.

The early editions give a wonderful insight into life in the 1930's. Each issue was full of news, photographs, profiles, advice on exercise as well as other areas such as political comment, letters and poetry, plus articles on a wide range of topics such as dress sense and family relationships, with the occasional recipe and a good serving of humour.

On the front page of each 1930's issue was the following information:

> 'The League was founded in March 1930, for business girls and busy women to enable them to conserve and improve their physique. It was started in the firm belief that pride of body is an essential foundation on which to build life and character. The rapid increase in the number of members seems to have justified this belief.
>
> The first exercise class to music was attended by 16 members in March 1930. Most of those Members are here today, which shows the lasting appeal of the work.
>
> The League started with a capital of £8 from Members' subscriptions. Now in 1933 each evening from 5 o'clock onwards, 60 classes in our London Centre alone are taken every week, not to mention the provinces and the suburbs.
>
> Stretch and Swing exercises for Health and Figure are taught; also Greek, National, Tap and Ballroom Dancing. The exercise classes last three quarters of an hour for beginners and one hour for the more advanced. Dancing classes last half an hour."
>
> Entry fee 2/6 Classes 6d. Experts teach the classes which are taken to music.

Large London business firms or persons living in the suburbs or country who are anxious to come in touch with the League, sometimes find it a problem to make a start. Just invite Mrs Bagot Stack to come and speak and bring a demonstrator; she will lecture anywhere in or around London free for the League, if her out of pocket expenses are covered and facilities are given for the enrolment of members after the lecture.

WOMEN, old or young, married or single, cultured or uncultured, you may JOIN OUR LEAGUE and become part of a WORLD-WIDE BIG IDEA.'

On the lower half of the page is a membership form which includes the following:

Dress: White sleeveless blouse, short black knickers. Stock knicker pattern available price 6d.

I promise on my honour that:
1. I will try as far as possible to acquire some practical knowledge of the mechanism of the body.
2. I will spend at least 15 minutes a day or one and a half hours per week on practical health-building, such as walking, running, or sport, in the open air, or exercise indoors with windows open if possible.
3. At night and in the morning I will think of and determine to acquire the healthy, fresh air body, which is my ambition.
4. I will do my best to co-operate in a friendly and helpful way with members of the League, and in the organisation to accept all rulings of the Committee.
5. I will try to introduce at least two new members.
6. I will buy at least one copy of each issue of the League Magazine, "Mother and Daughter".

The following advert was placed on the next page:

'A WORTH WHILE CAREER FOR GIRLS. Train to be a League teacher.'

Then all the current Centres were listed: In the Suburbs were:

Acton, 'Bromley, Croydon and West Wickham', Finchley, Finsbury Park, Golders Green, Ilford, 'Kew Kingston and Richmond', Perivale, Wembley and Harrow, Wimbledon.
In the Provinces:
Belfast, Birmingham, Bournemouth, Brighton, Glasgow, Liverpool, Manchester, Nottingham, Reading and Slough, Southampton, Southend.

VOLUME 1: NUMBER 1

In the first issue there were two articles by Mary Bagot Stack. The first was called 'Good Ideas' describing how she gets her ideas:

'How do you get ideas? I get mine in my bath! GOOD IDEAS are behind every successful venture. Members, part of this page will be kept open for your good ideas. ... LOYALTY is a very good idea. Loyalty to our friends our employers our colleagues. It unifies our actions. Loyalty to our League aim – racial health, physical, mental, spiritual – has unified our League and this has made it grow amazingly in three years. ....'

This is followed by the second chapter of her life story, called 'Romance of the League' in which she describes how she came up with the idea of creating the League, an extract of which is reproduced in Chapter One of this book, giving an insight into Mary's personality and thoughts.

In the first edition there was also advice on exercises for a better figure, reports of the previous years' League Week in Hyde Park and the Royal Albert Hall, and reports from the first major displays held by Centres in Bournemouth and Glasgow. The remainder of the journal contained a range of eclectic offerings. There was a short list of DON'TS entitled 'Education for Mothers' from her 'daughter'. Included in this are:

'DON'T be anxious if I am not in until 5 a.m.; and DON'T jump if I take the car round the corner on one wheel; it's quicker.'

Some things don't change!

Another article is quite different and clearly shows just how much other things do change. It was entitled 'How to Spend £5 wisely', that is, on a new wardrobe for autumn. It reminds us that 'no guarantee of good taste goes with tons of money', so a limited budget is set. Most of the items suggested are brown in colour and the main luxury appeared to be the hat.

'Now for the hat! Our biggest problem. Don't let us hurry over it; let us be sure we get one we shall enjoy wearing all the winter, a hat chosen in a hurry is seldom, if ever, a success. If we have saved some shillings from our previous purchases let us be extravagant and get something different.'

What becomes apparent in this article is that the suit and frock are to be home made, and the jersey to be knitted. So for £5 it was possible to buy the necessities for a two-piece suit for 14/9 (14 shillings and 9 pence); a jersey 10s, shoes 12/11, gloves 5/11, two pair of stockings 9/10, a hat £1, a frock £1 and sundries, clips, brooches veil or ribbon, 6/7. An explanation for younger readers: there were twenty shillings to the pound and twelve pence to the shilling.

Every issue had at least one political article. In the first issue this was about the World Economic Conference. This addressed the issue of how countries could regain the economic output and growth that existed in 1929, as the current economic climate was creating unemployment, starvation and misery across most developed countries. It noted that World Trade in 1932 was less than half that of 1929. Subsequent magazines continued this theme charting the political and economic lead up to World War Two.

Other articles explained how the human blood system worked, how to recycle waste, singing games for children, careers for daughters and how to look immaculate. In the article on recycling waste, written by a Covent Garden opera singer, no less, the waste is not passed on for recycling but put to immediate re-use. Banana skins could be used to clean brown shoes, pieces of orange peel can be scraped to provide flavouring, then used as slug traps, and finally dried and used as fire lighters. The sheer ingenuity of the 'waste not – want not' lifestyle is particularly impressive when set against our present day disposable society.

On the final page of the first magazine was a poem written by a member. In later issues there were a number of more romantic verses, but there was also space for the often humorous efforts of readers. Enjoy:

'ROUGHAGE, by Mrs Simpson

When indigestion tears your vitals,
Take no drugs with fearsome titles:
Waste not your gold on pale pink pills
For liver, spleen or kindred ills.

If your alimentary tract
With food unwanted is tightly packed;
And little Mary makes you cuss
And think of dynamite and wuss.

Or with leaden heart you dine
With one eye on your intestine:
Then take this remedy most kind
To cure your flatulence and wind.

A spoon of roughage – oatmeal, neat;
T'will set your stomach on its feet;
Your innards will digest your food
Behaving as good innards should.

E'en tho' it hath a gritty taste
T'will clear the crannies round your waist:
Tho' it resembleth gravel path –
It holds no dreaded aftermath.

So let not friend nor foe rebuff
But munch your oatmeal good and rough;
Then, swept and garnished – give the praise
To roughage – all your pleasant days.'

Equally illuminating are the advertisements carried; very few in the first issues but gradually building up to offer a range of products and services deemed relevant to the lives of busy women. Adverts for deodorants, cream to 'Banish Wrinkles', stockings, shoes, clothes, natural therapies, and all forms of cosmetics. There are many things that do not change.

The literary style of those days can be judged as far more flowery but there was also a certain elegance which is largely missing, today. The advertisement for the Pomeroy Original Skin Food explains that it:

> 'Bestows a triple blessing upon all who use it. The thrilling loveliness of youth. The cultured perfection of maturity. The well preserved lovableness of later years. What sweeter legacy could any women desire?'

The most unexpected advert was by Chapman and Hall who advertised 'Four Important New Books: Fit or Unfit for Marriage (by a medical practitioner); The Improvement of Sight by Natural Methods; Heredity-Mainly Human, and The Family: its sociology and social psychiatry.' The most unusual advert was from Winsor and Newton supplier of artist materials, offering a

> 'Bowl for graceful Walking Exercise, size seven and a half by three inches, for balancing on the head.'

1930's

The early magazines were a wonderful, if not unique combination, which both lived up to the ideals of its founder and yet never took itself too seriously. In every issue there were articles by Mary Bagot Stack in which she explained her ideas and ideals. She did not write about external beauty but on other forms of beauty, such as purpose, truth, loyalty and peace. In one article, Mary talks of how to reach ideals of truth and beauty and how the body needed to be sensitised to 'hear' or tune in to the music of truth that might inspire us to true actions. This she felt was the only guide to real knowledge.

An article in 1933 by the regular contributor, A.C.E. is entitled 'Fascism or Liberty?' It presented a comprehensive and easily understood account of a key political issue, the problem of Government. What might be the future of Democratic or Parliamentary Government, and whether it is the best form and can it survive? The failure of democracy in Germany and Italy was a great cause for concern. The article goes on to talk about the rise of fascism, and how it was 'OK' when it was confined to Italy, but since it has spread, how it posed a very real threat to the world. The journalist known only as A.C.E. wrote a political article for every edition. When he retired, the occasional article on social and political issues was contributed by Mrs Helena Normanton. Readers in 1935 would have recognised this name, as she was a prominent figure in the struggle to open the Bar to women. Mrs Normanton was the first woman to appear as counsel at the High Court of Justice, Old Bailey, North London Sessions and at the Bradford Sessions. She expressed sympathy with the ideals that inspired the League, and being in contact with many of the leading personalities of the day, she was deemed an appropriate person to offer independent and informed judgement on public affairs.

The articles on the history of the League, on health and fitness, fashion and book reviews continued. As Centres opened up around the world, regular reports were sent in to update everyone on a wide range of developments. Those members who had ventured out from the UK to visit far flung places, also wrote articles and sent letters. From the outset the magazine has formed a link between the UK and Centres throughout the world. Members continued to contribute articles, poetic contributions and letters, all on a wide range of topics.

Extract from a letter to the journal in 1934.

'Dear Editor, Can you help me? My symptoms became alarming after a particularly hilarious class taken by Prunella. We were taught a new knee twist to the vocal accompaniment of "All I Do is Dream of You". Well, going home, I could not resist demonstrating this new hop on the bus platform and gazing wistfully up into the conductor's face murmuring "All I do is dream of you". He was not much impressed and looked not only surprised but suspicious. ... In church the next day one hymn was particularly suited to "Wiggle-Waggle" and by the end of the last verse my spine was beautifully loose and I kept a beautiful waggle position but I was led gently out by the warden between pews of gaping congregation.'

NEW NAMES, NEW FORMS

By the autumn of 1935 the circulation of 'Mother and Daughter' had trebled. In November 1937 it changed its name to 'Health and Beauty', to reflect more closely the work of the League, and the circulation continued to increase. There was so much of interest in the League's early magazines that any member who has copies should pick them up again and enjoy a stimulating read!

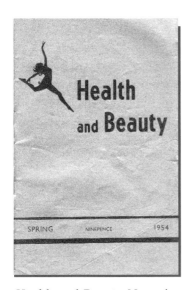

Health and Beauty Magazine

The magazine has continued to be produced in a variety of formats and with different titles, to the present day. There has been a need to keep pace with changing fashions and styles in magazine layout, as well as changing economic conditions, new editors wishing to reflect a different style, and most importantly attempts to ensure that the magazine remained relevant for its readers.

The unusual silver cover disappeared in 1961 and with it the famous logo of 'Peggy's Leap' from the front cover to the back. Different coloured covers and logos appeared with each issue, although the content remained broadly the same. The section covering the news from the Centres was expanded and this was a change welcomed by readers. Other changes to the magazine were debated in the readers' letters columns and in the editorials. Thus when, in 1963, the magazine had its price doubled to one shilling and sixpence, because of increasing losses, the readers understood the necessity of this and circulation did not suffer greatly. However in 1965, due to financial pressure, it was decided to drop the summer edition and produce just three issues each year.

The name of the magazine remained the same for thirty six years, until 1969 when it was changed for a second time to 'Poise', and a new format was devised. The page size was increased and the symbol of 'Peggy's Leap' was reinstated onto the front cover, which was otherwise plain white. More significantly the number of issues was reduced from four to just two per year, in the Spring and the Autumn. This innovation was short lived. The AGM held in 1970 reported that the magazine was a 'strain on League finances' and that there was an urgent need to increase circulation. Autumn 1970 saw the fourth and final edition of the magazine in its new format.

In 1971 the magazine was replaced by a Newsletter, called 'Health and Beauty News', which was to be produced twice a year. In this significantly different format, gone was the cover, and general articles and instead the Newsletter format put the editorial on the front cover, and limited the issues to be covered, to reports from meetings, teacher training courses, special events, forthcoming events, news from overseas and news from the regions. In some years the promised two editions emerged, but in many there was just the single issue. By the mid 1980's, the format had remained unchanged, but there had been an increase in the number of pages.

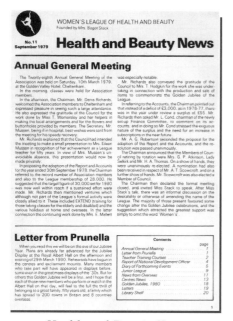

Health and Beauty News

Vicki Barter, who took over as Editor in 1976, retired in 1986. Vicki first joined the League in 1932 and performed in the Albert Hall display of 1933, and had contributed to several national displays. She was Prunella's secretary for the magazine as early as 1933 and typed all three of her books. After her retirement she continued to work for Prunella. Until a new editor would be found, Prunella stepped into the breech. By the second issue, Prunella was sharing the editorial role with Tricia Hodgkin and Joan Scott.

In 1987 there was another significant change as the name was amended to 'Health and Beauty Exercise', in line with the new working title of the League itself. The magazine was produced in A4 size for the first time, with a different design plus photo on each subsequent cover, but retaining a smaller logo of 'Peggy's Leap', and with just one edition each year, in the Autumn.

The demanding job of editor was taken over by Pat Sloman in 1992 and then by Caroline Quigley in 1994. Caroline has been in the hot seat ever since. In 1999 she oversaw the total 'makeover' of the magazine, although the size stayed the same, once more reflecting a change in name and management of the League.

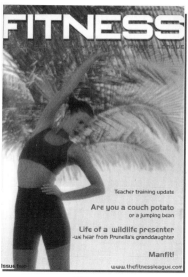

Fitness

Both shared the new title of 'The Fitness League'. However after only five issues, one or two each year, this new styling was in for yet another change.

The current League magazine is produced once a year, each September, and it is titled: 'FITNESS: the official magazine of the Fitness League'. Inside are the most noticeable changes with a greater use of colour and font size and type. This modern format maintains the range of interesting and relevant articles and it is available free to UK members. It continues to be a vital and valued link between head office, teachers and members world wide.

CHAPTER 6

THE LEAGUE OVERSEAS

In autumn 1930 the League began classes in Belfast and by the autumn of 1934 there was a new Centre in Dublin. By 1935, just five years after its establishment, the League had Centres in countries as widespread as Australia, Canada and Hong Kong. The League was to face new issues in setting up overseas, as other cultures responded in different ways to the idea of women taking control of their health and development.

IRELAND

It was a letter from a relative, Mrs King, asking Mary Bagot Stack to open a Centre in Belfast, that decided Mary on opening Centres in other parts of the provinces. Eileen MacMurray was a teacher who first met Mary in 1925, trained at the Bagot Stack School, and later went over to Ireland to join with Mrs King in pioneering the new Centre. Eileen had been teaching in London, but being Irish she was willing to return to her native country. She later wrote:

> 'Mrs Stack suggested that I should join her classes in London particularly as she wanted an Irish student. (Once the League was established) the idea of a Belfast Centre was put forward and Mrs Stack suggested the obvious thing was to have me as teacher. The League was literally launched on a sea of enthusiastic women and girls. First enrolments numbered five hundred and quickly increased to a thousand. My first class was so crowded that I could only take arm and head movements. I remained at Belfast until 1934.'

The papers were full of this news and this attracted a large audience to the first display and lecture, and the hall was packed. Mary Bagot Stack attended the event and at the end, she offered to teach a free class there and then! Mrs King, whom Mary described as a very young grandmother, proceeded to take off her dress and exercised in her petticoat!! When they asked all those interested in joining to stay, and the rest could leave, virtually nobody went. At the first class the queue stretched all the way down six flights of stairs and out into the street, all three hundred and seventy one members.

Establishing the League became problematic when the name 'The Women's League of Health and Beauty', was challenged by the authorities, as they disliked the use of the word 'Beauty'. Mary Bagot Stack sent a message saying 'Change the name, do anything, I know you will keep our ideals'. So to avoid any problems the name adopted was Ireland's League of Health. The use of the logo based on Peggy St Lo's leap was banned, due to her lack of modest clothing! The authorities also demanded that members should wear skirts over their short pants, when giving displays in public. By this time, in 1934 Kathleen O'Rourke who was a teacher at the Bagot Stack Health School, became involved in the new League in Ireland. It was important that the League gained the approval of the

Church as Kathleen was related to one of its senior figures Archbishop MacQuaid. He asked her many questions about the purpose of the League, before it was allowed to open. Essentially he wanted to know how their teachings and purpose corresponded to the teaching of the church. Ultimately, however, success was as rapid in Ireland as in England.

After the outbreak of war in 1939 only a few League classes continued, often running at a loss. Kathleen O'Rourke returned to Dublin at this time and took a job working for the Vocational Education Committee, taking exercise classes. Unlike any of her colleagues, Kathleen donned the League uniform and taught as if it were a League class. None of the students had experienced League methods before, and members of the class later told her that they thought her quite mad! In official League classes the focus was on the educational and health benefits, for children as well as adults, and the number of remedial classes was increased. It was also made possible for the League to conduct classes in schools, and colleges. In 1945 the Dublin Centre held a Theatre Show which included technical school pupils and students from the Gaiety School of Acting where Kathleen had been teaching. She remembered that one of the shows participants was a young man named Eamonn Andrews.

After the war Kathleen was invited back to resume her teaching at the Training School, but she declined because she was by now committed to reducing the League's debts in Ireland, and building up classes again. As a compromise she promised to return to London for six months in 1946 to teach a short training course. In 1947 Kathleen founded the Dublin College of Physical Education. During the 1950's much of Kathleen's time was spent working at a remedial clinic and running ante natal classes, but she still managed to fit in her League work, which she increasingly shared with Isolde McCullagh.

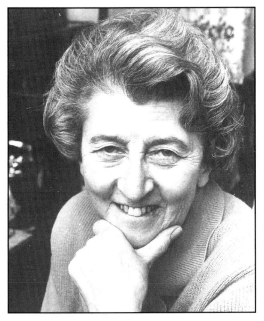

Kathleen O'Rourke

Over the years attitudes changed and the skirts were shed and the logo reinstated. Rallies and displays we held regularly and the League's development mirrored that of its sister organisation in the UK. For the 40th anniversary in 1974 there was a display at Shelbourne Hotel, at which Kathleen was honoured for all her work. Her health was failing, but she continued to do what she could until her death in 1980. In 1984 Isolde introduced EXTEND to Ireland which has gone from strength to strength.

The Golden Jubilee for Ireland was in1984, and this was celebrated with a big display in the UCD Sports complex. The League continued to open new Centres. Despite her own illness Isolde continued teaching and training new teachers. By 1999 the League was sixty five years old in Ireland and Isolde had been teaching for sixty years. The weekend celebrations brought so many visitors from the UK that there was no room left in the hotel for the Irish. Both Prunella and Pat Rowlandson, who had been the main examiner for the Irish teachers, went over to Ireland for the celebration.

CANADA

1935 saw the League opening in Canada. The 25th September was Canadian Foundation Night in Toronto and Prunella was there with Delphine Solon and Natalie Platner. At the Canadian National Exhibition preceding the opening, Delphine and Natalie gave eight demonstrations a day, sold six hundred magazines and distributed thirty four thousand leaflets. Membership of the League grew very rapidly. The success was such that the following year in 1936, they sent a team from Hamilton and Toronto, to England for the second Olympia display. They were the first team beyond the British Isles to send a team to a display in the UK. The efforts to raise money so that they could send another team in 1939 began the year before. Every Centre was working hard to contribute to the Wembley fund with bazaars, demonstrations, fashion shows, dances and ten pin bowling figuring among the multitude of events. The enthusiasm of Canadian members was clear, as a list of over sixty names were collected, of those who wanted to be in the next team to be sent to Wembley.

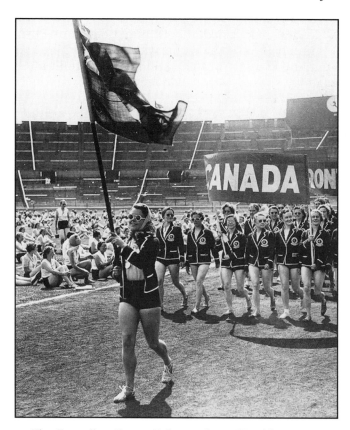

The Canadian Team, Rehearsals at Wembley 1939.

Early in 1939 an impressive looking legal document, covered in red seals and green ribbon, was received by the Canadian League, recognising the establishment of the League as a Canadian company.

By 1950 League classes in East Canada were being held in Toronto, Oshawa and Hamilton where there were now one thousand eight hundred members. The Canadians sent a group to Wembley for the UK's 20th anniversary celebrations, again with the help of raffles and collections; the team included eighteen members from Toronto, one from Oshawa and five from Hamilton. The youngest member was just nineteen and was joined on the team by her mother.

On the other side of the continent, in British Colombia, in 1950, Diana Kropinska was establishing a Centre in Ganges on Salt Spring Island, midway between Vancouver and Victoria. The opening demonstration was on the 23rd October, and two classes started the following week. The pianist was Mrs Warren Hastings who had played for the League initially in Tunbridge Wells. Diana later opened a League Centre in Vancouver and regularly brought teams to the Royal Albert Hall Displays.

1961 was the Canadian League's Silver Jubilee. There was a full week of celebrations planned and they were delighted that Prunella could attend. Prunella's plane arrived three hours early and there was no-one to meet her, and then, when someone did finally arrive, she was driven over thirty miles in the wrong direction. Prunella did eventually reach Toronto safe and sound! There were several radio broadcasts and television performances involving League members during that week, which meant driving many miles between centres, and in Toronto the League celebrations even made the main evening news programme.

There was another memorable event in Toronto in the summer of 1967, when about four hundred members from the UK went to Canada for League Convention. Jo Aldwinckle a Canadian member wrote at the time:

> 'They came in droves, three plane loads of them from all parts of Scotland, England and Wales and their infectious good humour sent ripples of friendship to the outer suburbs of Toronto. The visit was tremendously stimulating for the Canadian members. It made us feel that after thirty-three years of existence we now meant something in the League as a whole, and that we 'belonged' to the family.'

Ivy Cromer a member from Streatham wrote in the magazine:

> 'The Associate members of the League from the 'Old Country' certainly took the fair city of Toronto by storm. The whole campaign was organised and administered by Elizabeth and Sarah Mallett, both small in stature but big in heart, with limitless funds of energy and good humour. We flew in, in three waves. I was on the first flight, which for some typically British reason was called 'B flight'. We were the pioneers who softened up the population and smoothed the path for 'A' and 'C' flights! We halted the flow of Toronto traffic and subway clerks quaked, and bus drivers

blanched at our coming. I'm sure the tale will go down in posterity of how late one evening a wise cracking driver transported a horde of laughing, white bloused Amazons, filling all the seats on the bus as well as 60 standing passengers! We came, we saw and – we were totally disarmed by the hospitality and friendliness of the citizens of Toronto. We all returned enriched by our experiences with new friendships forged.'

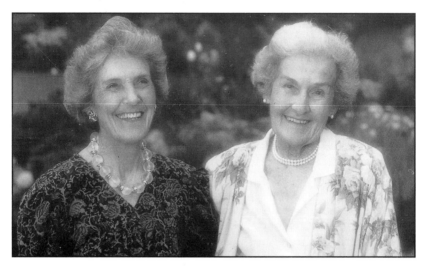

Diana Kropinska with Prunella, Vancouver 1993.

1993 was Vancouver's 25th Anniversary. Prunella attended and eleven teachers took part with two items, 'On Show' by Linda Spray and 'Antarctica' by Margaret McAllister. There were also visitors from South Africa and New Zealand. A hectic weekend was finished off with a relaxing cruise around the Vancouver shoreline on the Sunday.

AUSTRALIA

The League was introduced into Australia in 1935 by Thea Stanley Hughes who trained in London under Mrs Bagot Stack. On her move to Australia she became the founder and director of the League there. The word 'Beauty' was dropped from the name, and the focus was placed on the remedial side of the work. In the first ten years there were six training courses held and centres had opened across the continent, including classes for junior members.

Throughout the early decades the Health and Beauty magazine was sent to Australia and each copy was circulated around members at the main centres. Thea worked very hard to maintain the high standards set by Mary Bagot Stack and she was not afraid to recall teachers for refresher courses and to close down any centre where she felt that the teacher was not up to standard.

By 1950 there were forty three thousand members in cities across the country. There was a particularly extensive timetable of classes in Sydney with up to eighteen classes per day, every day in the week and including Saturday mornings. The League in Australia did not hold displays, but they were very keen to visit the UK for the 20th anniversary.

NEW ZEALAND

One of the original graduates from Mary Bagot Stack's Health School, was Millicent James (nee Ward) who emigrated to New Zealand in 1937. Once there she introduced the League system of exercise under the name of the 'Health and Beauty Movement'. The first classes were held in Auckland and within a week membership had risen to over one hundred. Larger premises were needed, almost immediately, and a hall was hired. There was also a need to establish a training school to ensure the growth could continue. Two years later in 1939 membership was eight thousand five hundred. Throughout the League's history in New Zealand, its main centres have been in Auckland, and the classes have continued to attract all ages, from teenagers to senior citizens.

In 1956 Kay Hudson a UK teacher from Leicester, emigrated to New Zealand and became involved with the League training programme for athletes that were going to the 1956 Olympic Games in Melbourne. League exercises were valued as they assisted with muscle toning and joint loosening. Regular Rallies have been held each year which enable members to meet old friends and make new ones, and as in the UK, the culture of organising holidays for League members also thrives, with a regular annual weekend at Helensville.

Members from New Zealand have often travelled overseas to Rallies in Canada and the UK. For the UK League's 50th anniversary, thirty six members, eight husbands, a teacher and pianist, all travelled over at their own expense. They were very proud to march into the arena of the Albert Hall under their own flag.

Such visits were eventually returned when in February 1972 a group of UK League members and their families; sixty two members, thirteen husbands and seven teachers made the trip to New Zealand. This turned into a thirty two day round the world marathon. En route to Auckland the plane stopped over at Bangkok, and when they landed there, they were presented with garlands and there was a huge banner across the front of their hotel saying, 'Welcome to the Women's League of Health and Beauty'. The welcome at Auckland was no less grand, as they were met by two Maori members in grass skirts with whom they had to rub noses. They were also invited to a reception given by the Mayor of Auckland. Ruth Anderson remembered her visit fondly:

> 'The Demonstration was a joy. Excellent classes taken by Joan and Peggy St Lo and Sarah Mallett, massed items by combined New Zealand and UK members opened the programme. The rest of the display included a Maori dance performed by the children.'

1997 saw the 60th anniversary of the New Zealand League, and they welcomed one hundred teachers from the UK and South Africa. The founder Millicent Ward James was there to greet everybody. The Rally included a Maori item as well as those performed by the overseas teams. A highlight was the New Zealand item 'Moments to Remember'.

SOUTH AFRICA

The League did not become fully established in South Africa until Prunella gave her opening demonstration in the City Hall, Cape Town in 1951. Prunella lived in South Africa for six years from 1950 to 1956 and established the League among both the white population and the Cape coloureds. After just five months, there were six hundred and seventy European and one hundred and fifty non-European members. Barbara Keys came out from England to help build up and run the classes, and this enabled Prunella to take a trip back to England in the September for the UK's 21st Birthday reunion. Upon her return, the League in South Africa gave its first display, an outdoor demonstration which included an item by non-European members, which was well received by a mixed race audience. The next hurdle in the challenge to apartheid, was for Prunella to get passports and exit visas for the two coloured women chosen for the team that was going to the UK for the 1953 Coronation Display. Despite great difficulty and often uncooperative authorities, this was achieved.

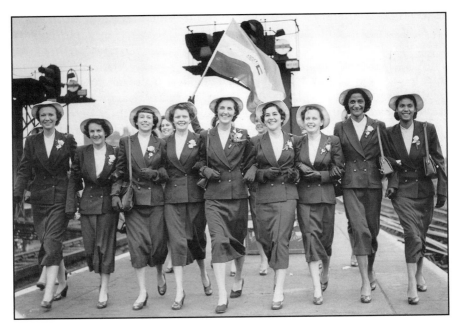

The South African Team arrive for the Coronation Display 1953.

Barbara Keys who had initially planned to stay in South Africa for just two years ended up staying there for life! She was responsible for the training of many League teachers, including Pikkie Smith. One of the members of Prunella's very first League class, Betty Bingham (later O'Donoghue), had trained at the Bagot Stack College, and she started the Johannesburg Centre in 1957. New Centres continued to be opened and the League grew in membership. In 1959 Joy Flanaghan took over the Johannesburg centre as Betty went to live in Cape Town and she was instrumental in opening the Pretoria Centre in 1961. That year was the tenth birthday for the League but all the arrangements had to be cancelled, as a state of emergency had been declared, following South Africa being declared a Republic. Fortunately the disappointment was short lived when later in the year a smaller celebration took place. It was not however until 1964 that the League name and badge was officially registered, after four years of trying.

South Africa's twenty first birthday in 1972 was special, as they welcomed Prunella to their celebrations. She returned again in 1976 for South Africa's 25th birthday, and on this occasion Prunella was interviewed on television. Joy Flanaghan also had an opportunity to appear on TV to promote the work of the League and she was shown teaching her classes in Johannesburg. As a consequence of these appearances there was a rapid increase in the number of new members.

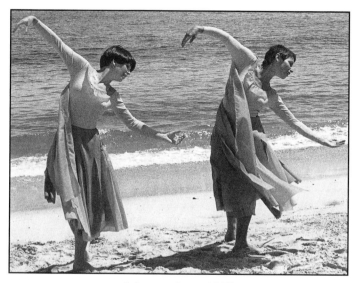

Johannesburg 1976.

The 40th Diamond anniversary celebrations, were marked by a large contingent of thirty two British teachers joining in the Display and enjoying the wonderful hospitality of their hosts. Their extended trip gave them an opportunity to travel round South Africa to other Centres as well as visiting Centres in Zimbabwe. There was also time off when they enjoyed a three day safari in Chobe Game Reserve in Botswana and visited Victoria Falls and Kariba. Cape Town's 50th anniversary was in 2002, when a group of ten teachers and members from the UK again journeyed to South Africa to present their items for the display. This was an especially poignant moment for Prunella, the guest of honour, as the founder of the Centre there.

RHODESIA / ZIMBABWE

The Salisbury Centre began in 1964, when Daphne Butler-Child a League teacher arrived in Southern Rhodesia. Before the end of that year a second course had been opened, held in the ballroom belonging to an ex Guildford member, Eileen Giggal. Attendance at all classes usually exceeded fifty. The League survived the political troubles of that decade despite petrol rationing where the individual weekly allowance was just six pints. Classes continued only because members shared petrol but they still needed to cram six or seven people into a single vehicle! Another problem was that it became illegal to send money out of the country, and this made it impossible for the members to buy the League magazine. Letters were sent to the UK asking if any copies could be given to them. Overall membership had grown to well over a hundred by 1973.

In 1980 the political situation was resolved and the country officially took on its name of Zimbabwe. Membership began to increase again, once petrol rationing was brought to an end. This led up to a very important celebration in 1985 as the League marked its twenty first birthday.

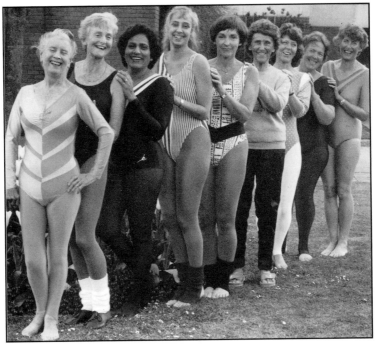

Teachers from Zimbabwe at a Refresher Course in the UK 1990

TRAVELS ABROAD

From the earliest days when Mary Bagot Stack and Prunella travelled around Europe seeking to learn more about different exercise regimes, many members of the League have enjoyed an opportunity to travel all over the world.

The secretary to the Executive Committee, a Miss E Ashburner visited the League Centres at Toronto, Ottawa and Hamilton, and was in Toronto in 1939, when news that war had been declared reached them. As she noted, the support and sympathy offered, brought home to her the proof of the League's will for peace, and the strength of the bond between nations and between women all over the world.

Individual League members who travelled widely could be found taking exercises classes whenever the opportunity presented itself, although by their nature these were temporary. One particularly intrepid traveller was Leonora Pitcairn who travelled extensively during the late 1930s and 1940s. As she wrote in 1947:

'Whatever the conditions we held classes – sometimes with only one person and myself- and sometimes with so many that I could hardly control them. Some might say that our classes were perhaps not worthy of the name but they had a character of their own.

My first classes in Africa were held in 1938 in a place called Jos, in the hills of Northern Nigeria. I began with about a dozen European women and soon we were nearly fifty. After six months I chose nine of them to do a simple demonstration to a large gathering of African ladies and the following week I began my African classes. They grew rapidly and the enthusiasm was splendid. We did a demonstration for the Governor of Nigeria and I trained six African women to take practice classes.'

When war came Leonora followed her husband to East Africa, but by the time she left Nigeria, there were mixed classes of Africans and Europeans and many of the exercise routines were being practiced to local African music. Quite remarkably she also gave classes on board the Dutch East Indies ship on which she found passage for the month long voyage. The music was supplied by a young man on his recorder! He had to find a position to sit, whereby he could only see Leonora, because watching the class caused him to laugh so much he could not play! Their ship was in a convoy with twenty four others, and, as she wrote:

'Our convoy was escorted by the 'Repulse' and we held classes every day at 10.30. It soon became noticeable that the 'Repulse' sailed close to our ship every morning at 10.30 and gave us a great deal of attention for at least half an hour. Everyone teased me about this but I didn't really believe we could be seen clearly from another ship and was amazed and amused when we reached Cape Town to be told by a young officer from the 'Repulse', whom I met, that they had enjoyed our 'swinging waists' the best! They had seen us perfectly with their glasses. I like to think they had a little passing fun over our class because they had little enough fun in their lives at that time and it was very soon after that we heard the 'Repulse' had gone down.'

Waiting a week for a ship to Kenya, she joined in classes in Durban. On arriving in Kenya she joined the army and was not allowed to hold classes. Instead she had to suffer army PT every morning, although this did not stop her from doing her own exercises in her cubicle at night. All routines were interrupted by the birth of her son Ian, after which her doctor insisted she have massage and take an exercise class. Leonora said she would accept the massage but would do her own exercises. The masseuse was very unhappy at this refusal as she felt that her exercises were the best as they were based upon those taught by Prunella Stack. This was a very unexpected but happy coincidence.

After a few weeks Leonora had to travel up the Nile with a small baby and sixteen trunks, to Cairo, to join her husband. This journey proceeded by boat, train and lorry. In Egypt she had to work and only had the opportunity to hold impromptu classes by the main swimming pool. As she concludes:

'I'm afraid members of the League would not think much of such casual classes but my hope is that many of these pupils will by now be attending proper classes in England. I wanted to let you know what fascination Health and Beauty held for people in all sorts of places and circumstances. How pleasant are our lovely halls in England and how delightful to bend and stretch to first-class music! But our unorthodox League classes had their charm too – a special charm of their own.'

Throughout, whenever League teachers have journeyed abroad League classes have materialised a short time later. A permanent League Centre has never been established in the United States but many members who have lived there have continued with their own exercises and run classes, and many copies of the League magazine cross the Atlantic to keep them in touch with the League. In 1955 Joy Flanaghan, a League member then working in New York, wrote about her experiences:

'I have now been working at the YWCA in Rochester New York for five months. My duties as one of the staff on the Health Education department are varied and include work in different sports, teaching swimming to the Rochester School for the Deaf, Volley Ball instruction and Tumblings and Trampoline on a Saturday morning for children. In my own field of work I teach tap, ribbons, health exercises, and a posture class for children. Right from the word 'go' women took to League work and numbers are increasing weekly. Public commitments included a most exhilarating TV interview and demonstration in which Ruth Anderson joined me and which to our mutual horror had to be performed in black tights, with our pants and blouses. Nothing Ruth or I could do, would alter this for apparently, tights had to be worn in case of complaints from viewers on the brevity of our outfit! This, coupled with the fact that our pianist was snatched from under our noses just before our demonstration – due to Union employment regulations – only served to spur us on to greater efforts.'

In the 'Land of the Free' the restrictions in 1955 were far greater than those in the UK in 1935!

This pattern has continued; one of many examples is Lucy Martin who in 1976 moved to Dubai for two years, and in less than a year she was able to report:

'We have a membership of over one hundred and forty, with sizeable classes of regular, enthusiastic attenders with whose progress and standard I must admit to being very pleased. I am also delighted with the number of nationalities represented, from Indonesian, Trinidadian, Italian, German and American.'

With classes being held in temperatures of 110 degrees Fahrenheit, this was quite an achievement. There were no Arabs in Lucy's classes because of the restrictions they faced with regard to clothing. In addition to this Lucy took hospital classes which led to her recording a set of eight exercises to be shown on TV as part of an Arabic medical programme. She was also invited to teach a class to nurses in training at the local hospital.

In 1978 another teacher, Rosemary Barber, went to Houston Texas with her husband. There was a strong British community there associated with the oil industry. Before long she had a toddler group and an adult evening class in a local recreation centre, against very stiff competition from aerobics, dancing, tennis and swimming. Rosemary also noted that women in America seemed far more reluctant to go out in the evenings, than those in Britain. At about the same time, Everett Harvey set up League classes in Kalushi, Zambia, in a village made up of people of all nationalities. In a very short time she had two classes running, and was lucky enough to have three former League members from England, living in the area!

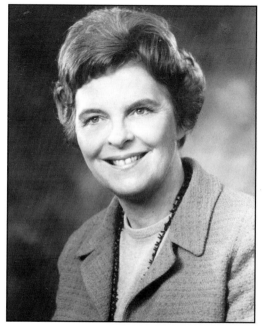

Elizabeth Mallett

The trend for League members to travel abroad to join in Displays continues to thrive. From the early days there has been one person at the centre of the organising and that is Elizabeth Mallett. Although in the year 2000 she retired from her role as 'travel agent', even after sixty years as a teacher, she continued with teaching.

The feeling reiterated by all those members who have been on League trips around the world is summed up by one member who said:

> 'One of the pleasant things about being a member of the League is that wherever one goes there is sure to be a fellow member and a friend.'

Across the decades the tremendous enthusiasm of members for these trips because of the joy and friendships that they bring, unites everyone. It is interesting to note the repeated comment that wherever they went they felt that what they shared with their hosts greatly outweighed any differences. At the centre of this feeling the most unifying bond was the shared ideals, and principles that first inspired Mary Bagot Stack. Her dream of peace and understanding between nations lives on.

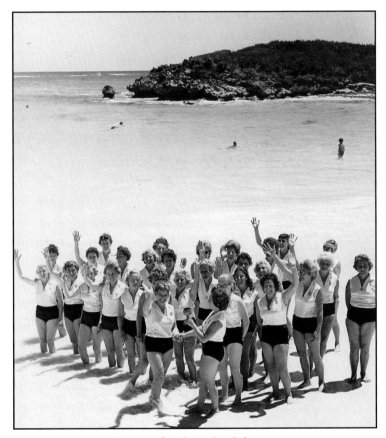

A wave for those back home.

CHAPTER 7

THE DISPLAYS

HYDE PARK AND THE ROYAL ALBERT HALL

The first public event held by the League was in Hyde Park in 1930. By that summer there were already over one thousand members, but Mary Bagot Stack realised that for continuing rapid growth they needed 'spectacular publicity' and without funds, advertisements were not an option. That was when she had the idea to hold a rally in Hyde Park, marching and exercising to the music of a military band. For this she had to get permission from the First Commissioner of Works, the Rt. Hon. George Lansbury. Mary took with her a photograph of a rally held by the Sokol movement in Czechoslovakia showing fourteen thousand people exercising together, to show him what the display might look like. Instead of a business-like official, she found 'a fatherly, rosy cheeked smiling old gentleman' who upon hearing her request said 'Of course you can have Hyde Park – Hyde Park is for the people.'

Mary also met with the Superintendent of Hyde Park, Mr Hay. When she apologised to him for giving him so much trouble he replied 'That's all right Mrs Stack, we are used to all kinds of cranks here!' Several newspapers had printed articles announcing the forthcoming display, so nervous anticipation was running high among the teachers and members alike. More good fortune came Mary's way when she was able to get the band of the Queen Victoria's Rifles headed by Captain Selth, to provide the music. Some of the newspapers had said there would be a thousand women but this was a little optimistic as not all members could attend. Instead there were about a hundred. Nevertheless the crowds came. Afterwards, George Lansbury wrote to Mary, 'This brings a thousand congratulations. It was just splendid; the girls looked healthy and beautiful. I am very glad my department gave you a chance. If you want to give another show later on, ask. Best wishes.' And so a tradition was launched.

Another League tradition is for major displays to be held at the Royal Albert Hall. From the earliest years of the League, to the present day, the Albert Hall has been the main venue for the displays celebrating important anniversaries. It was only in the mid to late 1930's when membership was at its peak that the Albert Hall was not large enough to contain all those who wanted to participate, that Wembley, Olympia and other venues had to be used.

The very first Albert Hall production was in May 1931. Teachers and members of the League were rehearsing as often as they could and Mary was struggling to find enough time to do everything that needed doing. However as she wrote of that time:

> 'Hard work, but I was very happy! I soon realised that production is what I like best in the world. The rhythm, the lighting, the music, the mass movement of large numbers was intoxicating.'

She continued, reflecting on the performance that night:

> 'I feel sure we looked very funny (the mixture of shapes alone would ensure that!), although we felt so almighty sublime! Humour is a fine quality, even finer, I think, than courage, for in its highest form it always has the touch of heroic in it. There is no room to describe all the happenings that night – the Graceful Walking Competition, the lights, the music, Marjorie Duncombe's beautiful nature rhythm 'The Forest', and Peggy St Lo's Tap Chorus.'

Could anyone on that day have imagined that this was to be the venue for major displays for the next seventy five years?

The following year saw the second Hyde Park Demonstration but it was not until May, 1932 that the second full League Week was held. This comprised the by now familiar Hyde Park venue, the march down Oxford Street, and the second Albert Hall Display. Prunella recorded her memories of the March and Hyde Park Display, in the League magazine:

> 'For months we have been asked: "What will you do if it rains?" We have replied: "Rain on the day of our Hyde Park Demonstration? – It just never does." We laugh, we sing, all self-consciousness forgotten. This is fun. It is thrilling to swing along through the park, thrilling to look back and see a long column behind us. Mrs Stack is leading us. Is she proud of us? Does she think we are doing our League credit? She looks as if she were having the time of her life.'

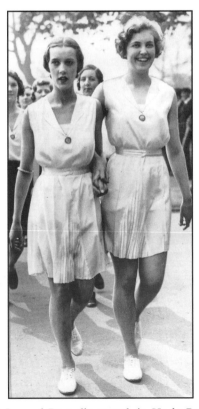

Peggy St Lo and Prunella march in Hyde Park: 1932.

First there was a speech by Mary and then the display. Once over, the performers:

> '.. burst forth into an hilarious three minutes of laughter and song, culminating in cheers for anyone and everyone, and then the triumphal exit, with banners flying and proud voices ringing out. The Hyde Park Show was over.'

On the following day the sun was still shining and it began early with a service at All Souls, Langham Place. After lunch six hundred members marched down Upper Regent Street, led again by Captain Selth and the band of the Queen Victoria's rifles. They were singing and marching, laughing and talking as they went. When they reach the Albert Hall Mary was standing on the steps ready to welcome them. Everyone raised a cheer. The profits that were taken that day were given to the British Legion Fund which helped unemployed men set up in business for themselves. This was seen by Mary as a way of helping people who had faced 'hard luck' and enable them to develop themselves through hard work. On a large and small scale so many of the League's events were used to raise money for other causes; another worthy tradition that still continues.

The format was repeated in 1933. In Hyde Park five hundred members performed to an audience of thirty thousand people, and the evening show was again at the Albert Hall. This was the first show in which representatives from Scotland participated, and Prunella produced a finale symbolising 'Peace'. A member from Glasgow, Betty Wright, wrote of that day:

> 'At first it was all just fun – glorious fun, to rush out of the Albert Hall with bare arms and legs and see the policeman hold up the traffic for us: we felt really someone then. Fun to march through Hyde Park with people taking snap shots of us; but as we got nearer it seemed to be something more than fun. One just felt it creeping up one's spine – that tremendous thrill which burst forth like a flame when we heard our marching song. At night came the performance in the Albert Hall. It just all seemed a sort of dream, a mad kaleidoscope of colour and sound and rush and excitement and a terrific thrill when the piper came in leading the Scots girls. And then the Finale, with the girls coming in and in, and in, and the marching song growing louder and louder, till all the hopes and fears of the past weeks seemed to blend together in one vast rush of enthusiasm.'

On the occasion of the fourth Albert Hall Display in 1934, the hall was taken for two nights running and every seat was sold. On the first night the items were performed by the League's suburban Centre members and on the second night by members from the rest if the country. The majority of the choreography for the displays was the responsibility of Peggy and Joan St Lo. Their creativity seemed endless and they seldom looked to other teachers or outside of the League for further inspiration. As the displays became larger, however, League teachers increasingly contributed items that they had choreographed themselves.

OLYMPIA AND WEMBLEY

In 1935 it was not possible to hire the Albert Hall as the planned date clashed with a Command Performance, ordered by the King, for Empire Day. So it was that the League went to Olympia, as the Grand Hall could take an audience of eight thousand. The event was still preceded by the usual Hyde Park Demonstration. Mary Bagot Stack had dreamt of a time when the League would be too big for the Albert Hall and all involved felt an enormous sadness that she did not live to see it. Everyone associated with the League wanted to make this event extra special as a tribute to the memory of their founder. Prunella asked many more members to join the march to Olympia so that there would be two thousand five hundred instead of the one thousand of the year before. As she wrote:

> 'This years' demonstrations must be the best ever and with magnificent numbers. Though only advanced and medium girls can perform in the shows, EVERYONE can join in our great recruiting march into Olympia. We want the youngest, and the oldest, fattest and thinnest, most elementary and most veteran, marching side by side.'

The march was so long that they needed two bands instead of just one. And at the Albert Hall, the Finale was a specially choreographed piece by Prunella, Joan St Lo and Marjorie Duncombe, as a memorial tribute to Mary Bagot Stack.

The first League contingent to come from overseas, a Canadian team, were welcomed to the 1936 Olympia Display. Three demonstrations were given by a total of over five thousand members and teachers, with a memorable item performed by one hundred child members. Continuing growth and success meant that in 1937 an even more ambitious display was planned for the Coronation Pageant with all five thousand members exercising together in Wembley stadium. Teams took part from two hundred and forty British Centres, which included Ireland, Scotland and Wales, as well as teams from Canada, Hong Kong, New York and Denmark.

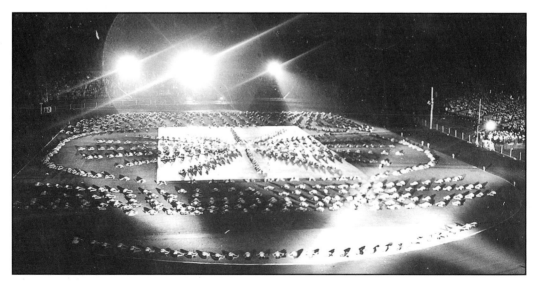

Wembley Stadium 1937

The enormous amount of effort and energy needed to continue to produce a spectacular show every year, was testing the stamina of even the most enthusiastic members and teachers. With a large show planned for the following year, it was decided that there would not be a display in 1938. The Empire Pageant of Health and Beauty, was held at Wembley with five thousand members in June 1939, and was produced by Prunella and Peggy and Joan St Lo. It was not until fifty years later, it came to light that taking part in the display was the then unknown author Catherine Cookson. In a letter she wrote to a League member, Kate Coulton, in 1988 she said:

> 'The fact that you are in the Women's League of Health and Beauty revives old memories. I was a member of one of the early groups, set up in Hastings; and I recall with horror the day we went to Wembley to join hundreds of other groups in a demonstration. Whether or not it was because I was such an individualist or I had no sense of co-ordination, I could never or would never keep in time with the others. And lying on my back in the great Wembley stadium I was petrified that I would be the only one to miss a beat.'

A team again came from Canada, and were joined by teams from Eire, Australia, New York and Hong Kong. Other members were welcomed from Bermudas, India, Jamaica, Malta and West Africa, as well as visitors from America, Denmark, Egypt and Switzerland. This was to be the last display on this scale.

With the onset of war, there were no further large League displays until 1946, when the first peace time rally and display was held at the Empire Pool, Wembley. One item was the 'Blues', which was remembered fondly by one member in a magazine article:

> 'Ruth Lane had suffered on our behalf, dyeing more than two hundred sacks blue, and dozens of others red. She had not been a lone sufferer, for Mrs Ormsby-Taylor had lent herself, her house, garden and all her pans and pails in the process. I understand that the dog also became involved and was a study in red and blue. To those non-Blue performers in our dressing room a word of praise is due also. Their frantic efforts to coax us both in and out of our costumes was a sight to behold.'

That display was held, like all others, with the only dress rehearsal having taken place earlier the same day. As another participant wrote at the time:

> 'Never would I have believed that anything could finally evolve with such clarity and precision after the dress rehearsal we had. Having rehearsed separately and in comparatively small halls, the result on the morning of the show was depressing in the extreme. The entrances and exits became more and more disorganised at every attempt, and due to the echoing of the stadium the music became a blur in the background, leaving us to struggle along on our own. The Production Committee exercised admirable patience and self-control, calling out instructions through the 'mike' encouraging us no end with their smiles and occasional jokes. By 6.30 the public were coming to its seats and suddenly it dawned on us

that these people were anticipating an enjoyable show and were looking to us to give it to them. Mentally we pulled up our socks and literally our pants and determined to do our best.'

For the League's Twentieth Birthday Festival, in May 1950, the display was held at Wembley with just one thousand six hundred members taking part. Only two overseas teams joined in, the ever faithful Canada and Ireland. The membership numbers never again reached their pre war levels and this was to be the last time that the League held their display in either of these venues, but in the years that followed, League members did perform there again when invited to rallies and shows organised by other bodies.

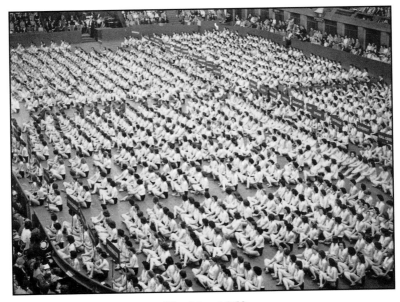

Wembley 1950

DISPLAYS FAR AND WIDE

The League continued to hold major displays in London to celebrate anniversaries and birthdays but hundreds of displays were also held around Britain by Regions and Centres, to celebrate their anniversaries and other local events.

The first held by the Birmingham Centre was in 1933 at the Wolverhampton Floral Fete. This was then the largest flower show held in the Midlands and was attended by thousands of visitors. Towards the end of that year the first branch display was held in Birmingham. The following year the League was invited to give demonstrations at the Brighter Homes Exhibition held at the Bingley Hall in Birmingham.

The Liverpool centre had their first demonstration in the Philharmonic Hall in June 1933. Olive Nevett wrote of it:

'I spent every spare minute I had for days before, practicing until I thought I must have been doing it in my sleep. I was so terrified I would overbalance and spoil the whole thing, and I would never have forgiven myself for letting the League down, with fourteen hundred people watching us'.

The Manchester centre held its first major demonstration at the Free Trade Hall in June 1934. A local member described her feelings:

'The limelight floods the floor, the band is playing a familiar foxtrot, and then a perfectly ghastly thing happens. The carefully rehearsed and memorised sequence of exercises takes wing and flies. In a dream I do various things which everybody else seems to be doing, then suddenly we all turn, amid tremendous applause again and march out. Have we finished? What a relief! Bad attack of stage fright. I spend the next ten minutes blandly informing everyone that, personally, I had enjoyed every second of it. And when next I take the floor I am agreeably surprised to find that I do. Then in a pool of changing, coloured light, two graceful, lovely figures move in perfect harmony through a maze of intricate steps at bewildering speed. Thank you Prunella and Joan.'

Croydon gave its first demonstration in November 1934, and this was the first event organised by a London suburban Centre. The event took place at the Croydon Baths Hall, with the participants limited to just fifty, as dictated by the size of the hall. Many people who came to see the show were unable to get tickets as it was completely sold out. The occasion was recorded in the magazine:

'First there was the hustle of changing in the cloakroom, everyone strung up to Concert pitch. The exercises never went with such a rip before. Time just whisked by, running on and off stage until we got to the special sequence that Letty and I had worked so hard to perfect. Anyway we were delighted to hear that Prunella said she must teach it at headquarters if we wouldn't have her up for copyright, but our item of course, belongs to the League. After several more sequences there were claps and cheers from the audience and the whole evening was over.'

The first big rally in Scotland was in Glasgow in 1938 at the University Athletics ground. This event, like all those before them, was a wonderful advertisement for the work of the League and brought in many more new members.

DISPLAYS DURING THE 1950's

In 1951, marking the League's 21st birthday, the display returned to its original home in the Royal Albert Hall. The first half of the performance was dedicated to Mary Bagot Stack, following sequences which she had evolved, while the second half was an opportunity to showcase more recent work. Prunella returned to England for this event, representing the League in South Africa, where she had opened a centre in Cape Town earlier that year.

The Coronation Display in 1953 was held at the Royal Albert Hall and 1,200 teachers and members took part. It was described by the editor of the League magazine as 'The most exciting show that the League has ever staged.' The Scottish team performed to the bagpipes, and there was an item by the 'babies', forty three in total, ranging in age from twenty two months to four years, which stole the show. A Canadian team was welcomed again, aiming for the record of the most travelled League members. Prunella came from South Africa with a team of twenty eight, which included two non-white members; their inclusion in the team was intended to demonstrate the League's rejection of any form of apartheid.

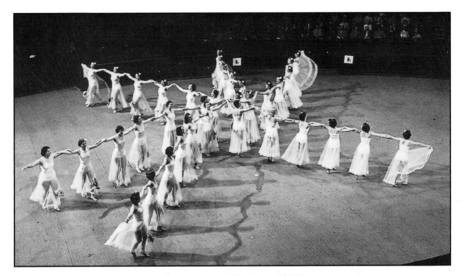

Coronation Display 1953

The main display of 1954 took place in Glasgow instead of London, where the Edinburgh team were celebrating their twentieth birthday. It was held at the Murrayfield Ice Rink and special trains were put on to convey members and teachers from all parts of Britain. This venue was selected for its size and not for the challenge of exercising on ice, and although the problem of slipping was avoided by the covering of the ice; this did not stop all those who had to sit on it or perform floor exercises from risking frost bite.

The 1955 Silver Jubilee Display was again held at the Royal Albert Hall, with one thousand teachers and members, representing all the UK League Centres, the Junior League and the Leagues in Eire, Canada, South Africa and New Zealand. This was the first major display that Prunella had missed, as she was at that time still living in South Africa. The 30th anniversary display was put on in December 1959, and attracted one thousand two hundred home and overseas members. This was the eighth display at the Albert Hall, and the sixteenth mass display held by the League, and the first year that a matinee performance was added.

COVENTRY CATHEDRAL

In 1962 the newly built Coventry Cathedral was to be opened. It was being built alongside the ruins of the old cathedral destroyed by bombs during the Second World War. At the opening ceremony on the 7th June, the Women's League of

Health and Beauty was honoured by being asked to perform. This event was unique in the history of the League. It had been over five hundred years since dancing had been permitted in an English church and now the League was to develop a ballet which would be performed in front of bishops and to organ music, and in front of a congregation from all over the world.

In 1960 when this possibility was first discussed the Provost had said that anything which took place that day had to be 'perfect'. 'Perfection' became the theme for the day. The League duly submitted a proposal, and discussions continued. The ballet was created to represent the transition between the different 'moods' as the Cathedral moved from destruction to rebuilding and finally to its Reconsecration. The Precentor suggested the music and the hard work began. The music had to be recorded both in a piano and an organ version, by tape and gramophone record, so that Peggy St Lo could create movements that fitted.

Peggy devised a three part ballet to the music of Bach, which was a series of short dance exercises to represent the three stages, entitled Anxiety (stress and despair), Faith and Joy. The costumes were professionally designed and made, and they needed to be suitable for a religious ceremony as well as allowing the performers the necessary freedom of movement. The costumes were scarlet and black for Anxiety; silver-grey for Faith and white and gold for Joy. Kathleen Ward organised the event, and eighteen local members participated, from Birmingham, Coventry and Leicester. Kathleen recalled in an article at that time:

> 'There was one crisis weekend early in 1962. Peggy came to Birmingham to teach us the last part of the new work. The music seemed so difficult, we could not seem to follow the organ, it was bitterly cold, and Peggy was worried. Should we go on or give up? We decided to go on. The members were wonderful. No-one missed a single rehearsal through all those months; no-one grumbled at all the travelling. It was this basic team spirit that kept us all going.'

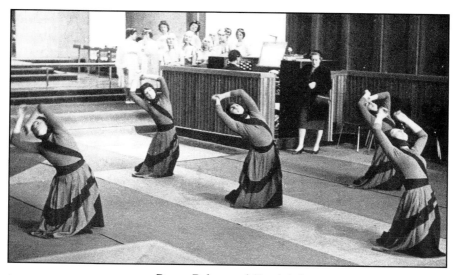

Dress Rehearsal 'Anxiety'

There was the first of just two dress rehearsals in the Cathedral itself in April. Instead of smoothing out many of the problems, it seemed to create many new ones. By May most of these had been overcome for the second rehearsal, which was held in competition with the constant noise from the workmen. On the 25th May came the actual consecration and Kathleen recalls her alarm at why they had ever supposed that they could make a suitable offering in this great new Cathedral; to perform on the shining black marble floor of the chancel before the high altar and the Graham Sutherland Tapestry. As she said:

> 'And so not only the day but the moment came. The performers were in their place fifteen minutes before the service was due to start. The great congregation was seated; the clergy and the Bishops had taken their places. The organist Mr David Lepine, played the opening hymn, the Provost made a speech of welcome; then came the familiar notes we were all waiting for... and with the actual moment came the inspiration of occasion. The eighteen members were no longer practising their parts – they were the embodiment of emotion; welded into a living harmony of movement and music which was thrilling to see and hear.'

This became the 'perfect' culmination of two years of preparation and nine months of intensive rehearsal.

Joyce Ellison, one of the performers, remembered the occasion:

> 'Oh what a joy to be asked to perform in the new Coventry Cathedral. Peggy St Lo has devised three items to describe the bombing during the war, next the end of the war and finally, the new peaceful beginning. The three groups were formed; the first was called Anxiety. Five members portrayed the bombing performing in black, with heads covered. There were bright red flashes in the skirts to depict the fire and destruction of war. The second item was Faith. Seven members dressed in beautiful silver grey satin designed to resemble a nun's habit. This routine represented the end of the war and the beginning of love and peace. The final item was Joy, which marked the rebuilding of the Cathedral and a new life for us all. This was performed by six members in white and gold satin dresses, with white and gold garlands in their hair. During the last few months the rehearsals took place in the Cathedral. The first sessions were held before the roof had been completed and we were amongst all the workmen hammering and shouting to each other. I was in the Faith routine and we performed to the music of 'Sheep may safely graze'. We had four beats in which to enter after the Anxiety group finished. When the music started, the four beats were kindly provided by the workmen, which made us all smile. We performed the pieces three times in the Cathedral and once again after, at another venue. Each performance was to a packed audience who had come from all over the country, and myself and all the other performers found this a very moving experience. It was a moment of which we were all very proud.'

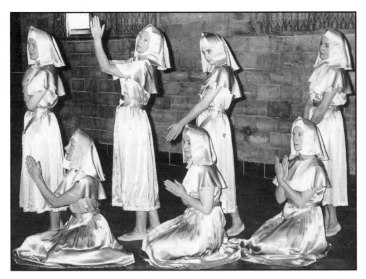

'Faith' - part of League ballet performed at Coventry Cathedral

As Kathleen concluded:

> 'The simple fact that the League was given this opportunity is something for which we shall always be thankful. We offered this ballet, not only as a personal gift from each one of us to this Cathedral, but also as representatives of the League to which we owe so much. Its triumphant success was a wonderful tribute to Peggy's genius, and to the splendid spirit of co-operation which Mrs Bagot Stack instilled into the League from the beginning, and which still inspires its members.'

Prunella came to the first performance and said afterwards that she had tears running down her cheeks, and even some men were moved to tears. Later that year on October 27th, the League gained permission to have a special service at Coventry Cathedral so that a further two thousand League members would have an opportunity to see the Ballet.

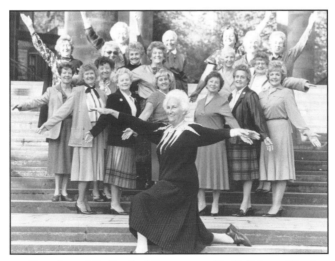

Reunion of Cathedral Dancers with Kathleen Ward
25 years later

THE SHOW GOES ON

The great number of displays held by regions and Centres over the next forty years are so varied and numerous that no summary can do full justice to the energy and enthusiasm which each has exhibited. Whether at Garden Festivals, in town squares, as part of other major festivals and events, or smaller local celebrations, League members have performed with precision and pride, in rain and wind, on slippery slopes and in mud, to audiences of all sizes. The benefit for the participants has been the satisfaction of a challenge achieved and the fun they have had; for the League it was a wonderful way to publicise its work.

A warm spring day in 1964, saw a group of intrepid members venture in the great park at Woburn Abbey. An invitation from the Duke of Bedford was not to be turned down, and the proceeds were for Oxfam. There were three hundred and fifty six performers, and a total audience of eight thousand. Memories are of an 'eventful' day when it poured with rain during rehearsals. The first display went fine but during the second the heavens opened again and completely undaunted, the performers continued through the final two items. When the rain started the Duchess of Bedford suggested they stop but when they carried on, she stayed with them by the piano. The event was judged to be a success and there was a return invitation in 1968.

Other regular venues included the Burma Star Reunions. The League was first invited in 1968 and went to subsequent events during the seventies in the Albert Hall and Blackpool, until the reunions ceased.

1970 was the 40th Anniversary of the League and as a break with the traditional Albert Hall Show, it was decided to have a Weekend Rally in Brighton at the end of May. This was organised by the London Centres and one thousand six hundred teachers and members attended. Joan Wilder wrote about it in the magazine:

> 'From the word go, the Weekend was an enormous success, no praise is too high for the London Committee headed by Joan and Peggy St Lo. The unique League atmosphere was created at the start by the four mass classes with four hundred members in each, on Saturday morning in the Exhibition Hall, Hotel Metropole. Prunella's class was honoured by the presence of the Mayor and Mayoress of Brighton. The Mayoress sportingly entered into the spirit of the day by taking her shoes off and joining in some of the exercises sitting informally on the platform. There followed an hour's delightful entertainment of a dozen items but space does not allow comment on all of these. But the gaiety of 'The Border Set' wearing tomato coloured jump suits in which three generations, grandmother, mother and daughter took part – cannot be passed over.'

This was followed by three receptions and meals at three different hotels each with their own list of speakers and guests. Joan, Peggy and Prunella were each the guest of honour at one of these. The next morning there was an open-air display on the Western Lawn of the Royal Pavilion given by the teachers and members from the Midlands, the North, Suburbs and Brighton, followed by an open class for anyone from the audience who wished to participate, taken by Prunella.

Never away from the Albert Hall for very long, the 45th anniversary in 1975 was just the excuse needed to return there. Over one thousand one hundred teachers and members took part in the display, joined by League members from around the world, and guest teams were invited to take part, from the Keep Fit movement and the Medau Society. Just two years later there was another excuse to retread old turf, when the League returned to the Cockpit in Hyde Park. They marched into the Park and performed their item during the Sport for All Weekend organised by the Sports Council.

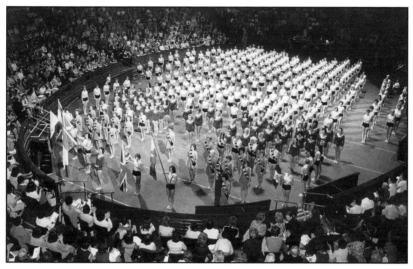

Entrance march 45th Anniversary Royal Albert Hall.

A very special occasion was the Golden Jubilee in 1980. Held on the 29th March, there were one thousand five hundred teachers and members taking part in front of an audience totalling ten thousand. A major rail strike had not prevented the performers getting to the Hall on time. Barbara Furniss and Bess Knowles chose and played a very varied programme of music accompanied by the Trevor Anthony Quartet. Onto the floor of the Hall were paraded the flags of England, Scotland Wales, Canada, South Africa, Zimbabwe, New Zealand, and Ireland. The ambitious programme had twenty one events, with special mention of Prunella's item 'tribute', for her mother. As the magazine reported:

> 'The First Sixteen, spotlighted across the arena, symbolised the small group with which the League began and two hundred and four members from the Thirties gained a standing ovation for their 'Swinging Waists'. The war years were dramatically portrayed and then one hundred and seventy teachers streamed on to the arena, ending their sequence by lifting arms in tribute to our Founder, a gesture reciprocated by many of the audience who rose spontaneously to their feet.'

During the Grande Finale, every member held aloft their gold covered programme and this sea of gold shimmered around the arena. Articles on the League appeared in over seventy five different newspapers and periodicals, and Prunella appeared on a morning chat show, while Seona Ross produced a short item for BBC's Nationwide.

Why wait for a big birthday? A return was made to Hyde Park and the Albert Hall for a Reunion in 1983, which was opened by a message of good wishes from the Queen. Yet again the Cockpit in Hyde Park became the focus, as Seona Ross wrote at the time:

> 'At 8 am the Cockpit looked cold, damp and miserable, and the cut, wet grass stuck to everything. Three hours later in the beautiful sunshine our miseries forgotten, we were reflecting on a wonderful experience. There was a terrific response from the public. Excellent taped music was the modern substitute for Captain Seth's Military band that accompanied us in the 1930's. The Run around the Park, nearly came unstuck when a public joker waving a huge umbrella persuaded the runners to go the wrong way. But eventually they all got back on the approved route! The classes which got off to a damp start finished in bright sunshine with a large crowd enjoying the infectious music. We even spied four policemen giving their version of a chorus line! The TV cameramen and the press were full of praise for the variety of work presented, especially when Prunella and her grand daughter joined in.'

The show at the Albert Hall mixed established routines with new. As Prunella commented at that time:

> 'In the second half special new items were shown, composed by Gloria Fear, Pat Jarnet, Lynn Wallwork, Denise McDowall, Margaret McAllister, Margaret Peggie and Carolyn Turner (now Kingdon). These illustrated the grace and expression which are two of the ingredients of the Founder's training. Their fluid movement, changing patterns and designs and modern taped music showed that the League is successfully adapting to the Eighties.'

The Diamond Jubilee in 1990 was again a moment to remember with its own unique atmosphere and joy. There were over one thousand four hundred performers and teams from six overseas countries Canada, New Zealand, South Africa, Zimbabwe and Holland, with an audience of about ten thousand. There were three performances, morning, afternoon and evening. In one item there were ninety mothers, daughters and grandmothers performing an item called 'Movement is Life', to show how the three generations can exercise together. The finale had an electric atmosphere with three hundred and fifty performers in the arena. This was an opportunity to celebrate the longevity and loyalty of League teachers, those with thirty, forty and fifty years of teaching behind them were given special appreciation. There were also seventy five members there who had joined the League before 1935, and for them there was a special presentation on the following day. As Liz Byrne recollected in the League magazine:

> 'The sunlight reflecting on the glass of the entrance lobby added an ethereal quality to the scene. Friendly ushers waited to guide us to our seats, progress through the labyrinthine corridors was slow, frequently interrupted by conversation with the many friends from far and wide gathered together under the vast, majestic dome. The lights slowly

dimmed, conversation gradually ceased as the atmosphere became charged with anticipation and suppressed excitement. What a splendid show it was! The opening item flooded the arena with vibrant colour, movement and life. The wide age range of the performers showed clearly that League work is indeed for all to practice and enjoy. For me, the children stole the show, they performed their items with well trained precision but never losing that all important sense of enjoyment and fun. The finale was the most incredible spectacle that I have ever seen and I am not ashamed to admit to the lump in my throat; the kaleidoscope of colour developing into a sea of glittering movement was a breathtaking sight.'

For the 65th Anniversary in1995 there were items from Canada, Holland, New Zealand, South Africa and Ireland. The League magazine asked new members to share their experiences of being first time performers. It is interesting to note how similar their reactions were to those of the first time performers of many decades earlier. As Irene Slack and Hazel Garner wrote:

'A rabbit warren of changing rooms, the incessant noise of chattering ladies, the heat, the colourful costumes! We changed on a spot of about two foot square and waited for our ten minute rehearsal. Before the first performance we nervously struggled into new leotards and tights. Our bras had been dyed in coffee to get the right shade, what would happen if it got too hot? We fought to control our nerves willing ourselves to enjoy the opportunity – the atmosphere was terrific and we felt on a high as we came off.'

Lila Masterman wrote:

'The rehearsal was held at the Albert hall and it was then that I realised how I was going to feel –TERRIFIED, absolutely terrified. However when all the girls got together it seemed as though something happened. There was such a wonderful feeling of friendship with people I'd never met before. Waiting to go on for the opening item I could hardly breathe. Suddenly the lights went up and WOW! I remember thinking 'I can't believe I'm here, my mouth was so dry that my lips were stuck to my teeth! The applause was wonderful and I sailed off the floor to the exit. I have never laughed so much as I did in the changing rooms, what started out so organised turned into utter chaos.'

The most recent show and one of double significance, was held in April 2000. Celebrating the new millennium and seventy incredible years, it included teams from South Africa, Ireland, New Zealand, Canada and Pakistan. The Sports Minister Kate Hoey attended and she spoke later about how very impressed she was by the fact that over one thousand members were so enthusiastic about the League that they were willing to commit the time, energy and money which taking part in the show involved, with many of them travelling considerable distances to do so.

The wonder of this show was that so little had changed since the days of Mary

Bagot Stack, with standards as high as ever. The Albert Hall manager remarked that the performers were better disciplined than the Marines. Not a rail strike but heavy snow, threatened to delay performers, but all went ahead on time. As with earlier displays there was an opportunity for the Junior League Members to show their skill and potential. Ten year old Rachel Tucker remembered her day:

'This was the most exciting day of my life! We got up early to get the coach and I was beginning to get really nervous when we got there. We were the second item on, the first item had finished so the pressure was on. As I was one of the younger ones I didn't come on at first. But when I did I was more excited than nervous. Near the end when we did the spiral I could feel my hair bouncing up and down as if it was going to fall out (but it didn't). At the end I started to enjoy it more because everyone started clapping. When we finished I couldn't believe I had done it, but I still had to do the Hornpipe and I had to do two cartwheels without falling over. We hid behind the buckets to start off with and then came out and sat on them. All of us were really squashed behind the buckets. At the end of the performance we knew our way round better than any of the grown ups.'

Given the League's remarkable history at the Albert Hall, there is absolutely no doubt that the celebrations in 2005 for the League's seventy fifth anniversary will eclipse all others in the hearts and souls of both the participants and the audience.

CHAPTER 8

TEACHER TRAINING

THE BAGOT STACK HEALTH SCHOOL

The first opportunity Mary Bagot Stack had to create a curriculum for the training of future teachers was when she opened her Health School in 1925. On offer was a two year full time course which covered: health exercises, anatomy, physiology, ballroom dancing, ballet, national dancing, Greek dancing, composition, mime, voice production, and public speaking. Mary was joined by two other teachers, Marjorie Duncombe and Dr Dorothy Dobbin.

All the exercises were carried out to music as this helped to harmonise mind and body. Popular music, including jazz, was used for the exercises and classical music for the dancing. The classes were graded from Elementary, to Medium and then Advanced and with each, the movements became more complex and improved the student's technique. The exercises were standardised and sequenced, so that they could be learnt 'off by heart, like poetry'. As Margaret Peggie explained, the students received a very varied diet of dance in conjunction with their training in health exercises, but it was the exercise system which was central to their teaching. When the students qualified they were able to begin taking their own classes.

In 1931, one year after the launch of the League, the school left Holland Park and moved to the headquarters at the Mortimer Halls. The teaching was still carried out mainly by Mary and Marjorie but they were now assisted by Prunella and Peggy St Lo, who introduced tap dancing to the curriculum.

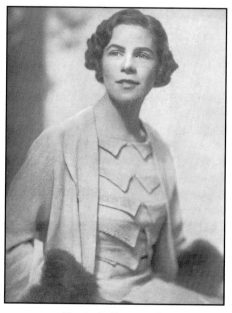

Marjorie Duncombe

In the advertisement placed in the early issue of the League magazine, then called 'Mother and Daughter', Mary tried to interest women in becoming physical exercise teachers, by stressing its wider advantages. She recommended that a girl choose a career that she would benefit from in the years to come. This career would make her 'a far more attractive and interesting person'. Not only would she learn to improve her physique and mental alertness, and to shoulder responsibility, but she would also enjoy working in a friendly and enthusiastic atmosphere.

The success of the League meant that the demand for places on the college's courses was increasing. By 1934 there were fifty students at the college. Once qualified, there was an opportunity to begin their teaching experience at the Mortimer Halls at a salary of four guineas a week for a minimum of twenty eight hours teaching. After that they became self employed, and were free to decide where they would like to teach, how often and for how long. Occasionally teachers were asked to move away from London and set up new Centres elsewhere. There was no compulsion in this but many did so because of the loyalty they felt to the League. One example of this, recollected by Margaret Peggie, was Betty Ayling, who was asked to move to the north east of Scotland to set up Centres in Aberdeen, Montrose, Inverness, Elgin and Nairn.

Many teachers continued in this role for the whole of their working lives. Others gave it up upon marriage. Although the League was instrumental in creating independent women with great initiative, there was still an acceptance that for some, marriage might come before a career. Marriage was what Mary Bagot Stack referred to as 'the final career'.

The School was closed during the war and reopened in 1946 at a hall in Ealing. There were seventeen students, seven of whom were on a special six months intensive course, which began in February and was designed for those with prior teaching and physical education experience. This course was designed in response to the need to produce new teachers as quickly as possible. The principal at that time was Kathleen O'Rourke who had trained at the physical training college in Liverpool. The curriculum changed, with the dropping of ballet, mime and ballroom dancing and the introduction of Medau Rhythmic Movement, musical appreciation, the history of the League and the production of Displays. Prunella recognised in the work of Medau, a holistic form of movement which complemented the exercise training of her mother. It was the movement training of the League that differentiated it from other major developments in physical education in the UK.

Several of the experienced students who had completed the first six month course, gave their views on the training in the League's Health and Beauty magazine. Mary Lillis told how she had met and been inspired by Kathleen O'Rourke. She admitted that she knew nothing about physical fitness and was initially wary, but Kathleen soon convinced her that through physical fitness she could experience a great change. Mary not only began attending classes but soon wanted to become a teacher. As she says of that first course:

'How shall I describe those six months? Months filled with sore muscles, dusty floors, tap shoes, café lunches (Oh! Those unsavoury rolls) and – scattered everywhere – loose bones – the skeleton's not ours! We became very intimate with that skeleton. Miss Wightman saw to that. She diffused among us a phenomenal amount of knowledge during her anatomy and physiology lectures and we are very grateful that we now share with her all the secrets of the Anterior Abdominal Wall. At first we wondered whether this abundance of technical detail was essential to our work but as the course progressed, the importance of this knowledge became increasingly clear. Every reliable pilot understands the mechanism of his plane and the right way to use it. The same should apply to us. The exhilaration of Kathleen's classes was great experience for us all. To her enthusiasm and intelligent interpretation of the work each one of us owes an inestimable debt.

As the days progressed we found the spirit willing; the flesh, alas, weak. Training the body in six months is a severe and sometimes hazardous task, but I doubt that students have ever laughed as well as we! It was Prunella who taught us the joy in the work, and during her classes to watch her move was an education in itself. Of the dancing, I would like to say that the classes given by Marnel King, Joan St Lo and Monica Curtis made a very real and popular contribution to the course. Apart from the joy of the movement, we all appreciated their kindness, their patience and their sense of fun. Just as the knowledge of colour and brush work does not create an artist, neither can the knowledge of the human body and the theory of exercise create a League teacher. It is all about the movement.'

Courses for others wishing to become teachers still required two years training. In total there had been sixteen students in 1946. In the first term, for example, the topics included Central Control, Head Poise, Elastic Breathing and Relaxation. Besides all the dance and movement classes held by the full time staff, there were many outside lecturers. They covered subjects which included training for childbirth, external visits, for example, to an experimental pioneer health centre and public speaking.

Summer Schools were run to give League teachers an opportunity to refresh ideas and to learn more. Just as importantly they offered a chance to meet up with friends old and new. The first Summer School after the war was held in August 1946 at Bognor Regis. This followed many months of searching by Peggy St Lo, for a suitable school in which to hold the event. Peggy eventually found a boy's preparatory school, and the bonus was that it was by the sea. Although the day of the teachers' arrival was grey and bleak, the following day the sun shone and classes were held out of doors. The lawn was shared by the students with several families of ducks! The teachers included Elizabeth Henderson, who had interrupted her house move to join the group. There was also Eileen Barnes who taught three new Tap routines, Marnel King who taught Greek and National dancing, and Miss Wightman who taught anatomy and theory of movement. Peggy and Joan St Lo arrived at the end of the week for the League general meeting. It was here that the Teacher's Association was founded, to help teachers to keep in touch with each other, share information and be informed of all League activities.

In 1947 a new training school opened in Dublin run by Kathleen O'Rourke, with just ten students, offering a three year course. The curriculum followed quite closely the range of topics covered on the London courses, but there were two items that were unique. The first was the Discussion Circle which met weekly to discuss art, literature and politics, and the second was the series of outside speakers on subjects such as taking care of teeth, social customs and etiquette.

THE BAGOT STACK COLLEGE

The Bagot Stack Health School continued with its pre war success, and was able to move back to Holland Park in 1949, to the house next door to the one in which it had originated. As student numbers increased the decision was made in 1955 to seek accommodation within a larger college. The renamed Bagot Stack College opened on the 3rd October, with Joan Wilder as its principal, based at the Morley College London. Non-political and non-sectarian Morley College was well known as one of the most important centres for non-vocational training specialising in the arts. Like the League, the college was founded thanks to the work of an indomitable woman, Mrs Emma Cons, over sixty years previously.

This was a significant financial commitment, and the Chairman stressed that there was a need to do everything possible to attract sufficient numbers of students to train, so that the League's work could continue. It was proposed that financial grants could be made available for suitable candidates. The course on offer was a two year diploma course in physical education for League teachers. The cost was £100 per annum and students had to be between seventeen and twenty five years of age. In 1957 Prunella took over from Joan as Principal, and Deidre Welsh joined the staff, just as the second two year course was about to begin. Two scholarships were then on offer by the League for suitable students.

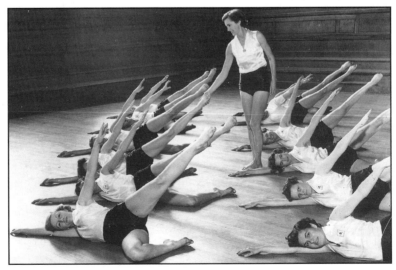

Prunella takes a class.

The Sixties saw the first ever deficit in the League's finances and the main cause was the cost of the Training College. With only seven full time students it became clear that more changes would be needed. League members responded with a series of fund raising events and in 1964 the fees were raised to £125. The Training College Appeal fund had by then just exceeded its target by raising £2,403 but there were still pressures on the League's finances. As the League depended upon a steady supply of new teachers, it was decided that the College must keep going and so the Appeal had to continue. £3,500 would be needed to complete the current course. By late 1964 the Training College Appeal had raised £2,326, but by early the following year the Council concluded that there was still a requirement for a further £2,000.

By 1965 the full time course at the Bagot Stack College was advertised as a 'Dual Course in Physical Education and Secretarial Studies.' The aim was to offer the student a wider choice of employment opportunities on graduation. Students were required to be between eighteen and twenty five. Fees remained at £125 and by 1966 the Training Fund had reached £4,000.

The 1968 course had nine students on it with one student, Solvejg Bording, from Denmark and one, Glynis Jennings, from New Zealand. Another student Jennifer Wolstenholme described the first time she went out on teaching practice:

> 'In the second half of our first term we went to various centres near our homes for teaching practice. Each one of us would do about five minutes of teaching on the platform to see how we felt about it and to overcome the shyness we all feel in front of a class of League members. Since then some of us have gone out in pairs to Centres without teachers and this has been the real test as to whether we can manage a whole evening's teaching and still have the members come back the following week. Well they did!'

In 1969 it was decided to introduce an intensive one year course at the Bagot Stack Training College starting in September, in an effort to attract more students, by reducing the expense they faced of living in London for two years. It was also the case that most students who had joined the dual course were only interested in the League training. By replacing the two year dual course where League classes were given in the mornings only, this allowed the students to complete their training more quickly. The syllabus included Bagot Stack exercises, theory and practice of teaching, anatomy, physiology, kinesiology, voice production and public speaking, movement and dance, and movement with clubs, balls and hoops. A new collaboration was set up with the College of Choreology, where students were trained in Benesh Movement Notation which originated in schools of ballet, but had been extended to all forms of dance as well as different forms of physical education. With some shared classes this gave the Bagot Stack students an opportunity to belong to a larger group of young people with similar interests. Many of the students at the College of Choreology were professional dancers from all over the world.

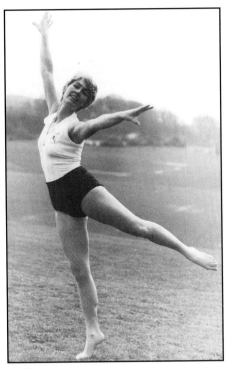

Newly qualified teacher
Margaret Peggie

With only five students on the one year course, financial constraints finally made the closure of the College inevitable. In 1970 as the students completed their course, this was the end of an era. As Prunella wrote at the time:

> 'The cessation of full time College training is sad, in that a chapter of teacher training closes with it. Many ex-students, now teachers remember their training days with affection and are grateful for the help and inspiration given to them by the College staff. The College has produced a cadre of expert young teachers during the last fifteen years. This has been possible because of the much valued help from teachers and members throughout the country, who have contributed so generously to College funds. But the League must adapt its training to changing conditions. Now the need seems to be for more widely spread, rather than centralised courses.'

Of the five final graduates, Leila Jaffer went to teach in Mombasa, Vicki Mason to Toronto, Karen Lake to East Grinstead, Maidstone and Tonbridge, Jane Roddis to Doncaster Leeds and Wakefield, and Julie Anne Smith to Kingston and Southall.

PIONEER PART-TIME COURSES

It was becoming increasingly difficult for prospective trainee teachers to participate in full time courses, in terms of the cost and the time required. For women with increasingly busy lives a new approach was needed if the supply of teachers was to be maintained. It was also seen as restrictive to maintain the upper age limit at twenty five. There were many older or married women who wanted to take on a new career, and so the upper age limit was raised to forty. The very first course was established in 1969 in the Midlands under Joan Jefferies. Twenty one advanced members had been recommended by eight Midlands teachers and they met in Sutton Coldfield on the second Saturday in each month for a day's training. These sessions ran from February to December, and if the students were successful they would qualify as Associate Teachers, and would work under the supervision of the fully qualified League teachers who had recommended them. This scheme had been prepared in consultation with officers of the Department of Education and Science, the Central Council of Physical Recreation, the League Council and the League Teachers' Association Committee. A grant from the Department of Education and Science was made available for half the cost of the scheme. Before the end of the year a second scheme was started in the South West under Elizabeth Mallett.

Joan St Lo visited both the schemes during the course of the training to ensure that the health exercise technique was in line with, and of the same standard as, the full-time syllabus of the Bagot Stack College. The part time course included a five day residential period, which was attended by both groups and all the tutors and teachers. This was a valuable time for friendships and discussions to blossom in the little time left for relaxing after an intensive twelve hour work day. Later in the course there were three residential weekends which Prunella attended. Following the success of this initiative, further part time courses were established, in Lancashire and Yorkshire in 1971, in London in 1972, and in Scotland and Wales in 1973.

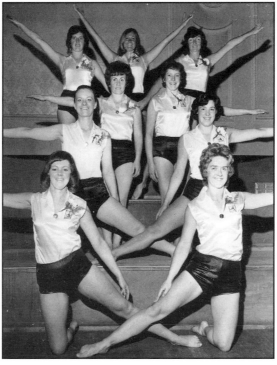

*Students from the first Scottish part time course
1974.*

In 1971 the first group of Associate teachers qualified, sixteen in the Midlands and nine in the south west. After setting up and re-establishing classes, this resulted in the recruitment of an additional one thousand members for the League. Approximately half of the Associate teachers decided to undertake the second year of training, to qualify as teacher-organiser. This training was run under the guidance of Joan Jeffries and Elizabeth Mallet and consisted of four weekend residential and two five day courses. In addition there would be eight half day sessions at Anstey College, Sutton Coldfield, with a final assessment in September 1973.

The Annual Report for 1974 records the growth of the League over the previous five years:

> 'The League has maintained its classes throughout the country almost unimpaired from the three day week and fuel crisis. Today it is poised for – appropriately enough – a big (and of course graceful) leap ahead. One of the reasons for this is the gratifying result of the training schemes completed during the years under review. The two year course in London produced fifteen Teacher-Organisers, the one year courses in Scotland and Wales nine and five Associate Teachers respectively. The success of these ventures has in turn prompted the organisation of a course in south west England. All this means that our teaching strength is being well maintained and indeed increased, at the same time as it is being rejuvenated. And a good supply of good teachers is the lifeblood of the League'.

PROGRESS AND CHANGE

Part time courses continued in many locations across the UK throughout the eighties with great success. In 1975 there had been a further forty new teacher Organisers and Associate Teachers and new schemes were set up in Leicester in 1976. The five year plan in 1977 included a training course in London beginning in 1978, one in Manchester in 1979 and another in East Anglia planned for 1980. By the late Eighties there were seven courses running.

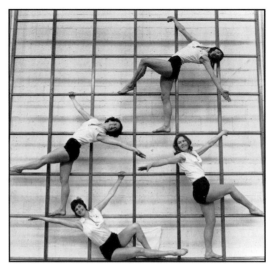

Teachers Lucy Martin, Rosemary Barber,
Margaret McAllister and Pamela Pickup at an
Easter Refresher Course

By the early Nineties it was becoming more difficult to attract new recruits. Given the very different market place for exercise in the Nineties, the Training Committee continued to adapt the training to reflect the changing expectations of the more 'exercise' aware society. In 1992 Margaret Peggie described the situation:

> 'Today the importance of making exercise an integral part of a lifestyle has become common knowledge so much so that in recent years a whole new industry has grown from this premise. It is important therefore that anyone wanting to train as an exercise teacher finds our courses as attractive and as accessible as possible. Without a continuing supply of teachers, the future of Health and Beauty Exercise is considerably at risk. To this end the Training Committee has as a priority the updating of our exercise system and the re-structuring of the Training Courses. We are aware that we must retain what is good and distinctly ours, which has proved so successful for over sixty years. Plans are currently being made for a streamlined more intensive course which will reduce the first year of training to Assistant teacher level to two terms or even shorter depending on the frequency of training. The second stage of training to Teacher/Organiser level will consist of series of modules, some compulsory, some optional which each student can collect at her own pace but within a given time.'

In 1993 two new courses were piloted with a more intensive training pattern, taking six months rather than nine to qualify as an Associate teacher. Also introduced was a new approach to the teaching of anatomy, kinesiology and physiology syllabus. A series of home study work books was produced by Lucy Martin, which the students completed, following practical classes in these subjects. The first pilot courses were sufficiently successful for a second round to begin. The following year these courses were fully assessed. It concluded that acquiring the skills needed to teach successfully took time and students on the short course felt that they needed more time for practice, to consolidate their newly acquired skills. As Margaret Peggie notes:

> 'There is so much to think about; demonstrating the movements on one side of the body while talking about the other, hoping that they fit with the music, remembering the coaching points, or at least what comes next, and all this in front of a sea of expectant faces!'

Margaret Peggie explained how streamlining the training course content to compete with other courses had proved problematic, and that the continuing success of the League depended on demonstrating the difference between what the League offered, compared with other forms of exercise. In this way she explained, the League would remain faithful to their conviction that the training and continuing support of the teachers must be given the time and attention it required. A longer period was again allowed for the first stage of the training. In 1995 Lucy Martin, a member of the Training Committee, took over its chairmanship from Margaret Peggie who moved on to develop her role in External Liaison.

In 1997 the training system for new teachers underwent more refinement as the length of Stage One was made variable dependent upon previous experience and qualifications. The course was designed to cater for students from different backgrounds, allowing more hours training for those new to the League system or with no teaching experience. Thus Stage One could take between seventy two and ninety eight days, delivered intensively in six weekends over six months or on single days over ten months. The full qualification would be gained by the new teacher obtaining the necessary modules over an extended period of time. The new style course made it possible to introduce it into Further Education Colleges and thus widen the possibilities for presenting the training. The course was offered as leading towards a National Vocational Qualification.

It was clear that the changes had been a success and new students continued to be attracted to the League's courses. The inclusive nature of the League's philosophy was highlighted, when a man was accepted onto a course being run in Cheltenham. Charles Reynolds was a university lecturer and a member of the British Psychological Society. He let it be known that teaching League classes was by far the most complex and demanding situation he has ever had to master. He is currently teaching in South Wales.

To attract potential new recruits in 2000, it was decided to introduce a Teacher Training Taster day, where potential new recruits had the opportunity to explore more deeply exactly what the course had to offer them. There would be participation in a League class, an exploration of the syllabus and a chance to learn about the Fitness League and its continuing education programme for teachers. In the latest League advert there is a list of qualities that a League teacher needs: 'A good sense of humour' is perceptively put as number one!

The age of those accepted onto training courses has also been relaxed over the years, with each student being taken on their own merit. By their very training League teachers have an exceptional level of fitness and energy and are capable of being both effective and experienced teachers long after any official 'retirement' age. At sixty five there is a formality that those that wish to continue teaching, write to the League for 'permission', but this is never in doubt!

Three new teachers interviewed in the League magazine in 2001, talked about why they trained. Teresa Moss was aged fifty three and a carer for the elderly who had learned about the League from a magazine article. She had no previous exercise experience but was determined to regain her own fitness and increase her confidence levels. She passed all her exams and now teaches her own classes. Anna aged forty had been a member of the League for ten years, and with her son at school she felt ready for a new challenge. With working as well, it was not easy for Anna to find the time, but perseverance ensured her success. Christele is French and had been a League member for six years. At thirty one she was looking for a more flexible form of employment as she planned to start a family, and she too is now running very successful classes.

The establishment of the Register of Exercise Professionals has helped to raise the profile of the League within the fitness industry. A review of the changes made to the training system brought useful information to light. Reducing the cost of the course by £200 did not attract additional recruits; and neither did extensive advertising. The analysis showed that forty per cent of students were relatively new members of the League; twenty per cent had been members for five years or more, and thirty per cent had some knowledge of the League. Just ten per cent were completely new to the League and most had discovered the training scheme via the website. With the setting up of a web page forty per cent of students are now recruited from outside the League and they have proved a valuable source of additional expertise and brought new perspectives to the League. However, there remains a strong basis of recruitment from within the League because of the subsequent high levels of success and commitment.

CHAPTER 9

THE MUSIC

THE HEART OF THE LEAGUE

Music is at the heart of the League's work. Exercises were originally carried out to the accompaniment of a piano, with music often especially written for the exercises. There have been many pianists who have worked with the League both in this country and abroad. Their versatility, dedication and artistry have been a crucial part of the League's history and success.

Music was important, not just as an accompaniment but as a means of teaching. The music was a natural partner to the movements and the two became inter-dependent. In some languages there is a single word for dance and song. Today in most exercise systems the 'divorce' between the two is almost complete. Without music, movement can be lifeless and inharmonious but when music and movement are not created to complement each other then the result can be artificial and unsatisfying. The League's use of music re-established the close connection between music and movement; it has been used to lead and inspire, and increase the rhythmic flow which required the minimum of effort and added to the pleasure. Music can awaken and strengthen a person's inner sense of rhythm and it is why the pianist accompanying a class needs to have an understanding of movement, rather than just provide a pleasant accompaniment.

The League required very special skills from the pianists it recruited, and for them not just to be able to combine the music with the movement but also to improvise. Not all classically trained pianists were able do this. However, there were many others who had less formal training but were naturally able to play music for movement. Whatever their prior training, the League pianist needed to possess an ability to perceive the dynamic of movement with the eye and then translate it into sound. The League was very fortunate in that it attracted several excellent pianists in its early days that could fulfil its exacting requirements. Most could play anything from Bach to jazz and could change tempo and style as required. Ideally the pianists in classes were in partnership with the teachers and, if not, then they needed to be led by the teacher as they would be by a conductor. Given the hundreds of classes held all over the country this was sometimes a very demanding standard to find.

The Bagot Stack School run by Prunella, Peggy and Joan, used to teach many forms of dancing and so they required a pianist that could play the widest possible repertoire. Not only that but they needed to be able to respond to the way that each class was being taught. If the teacher wanted to change the beat or the tempo, the pianist was expected to change style immediately. One of the many pianists based in London was Joan Ore who began playing for the League in 1934. She first accompanied classes in Cricklewood but then in the late 1940's began playing for the Training School. A pupil described her playing as expressing the movements perfectly, and being so infectious that she carried the class along with her. Deidre Welsh, also London based, was one of the foremost pianists in the early days.

DEIDRE WELSH

Deidre Welsh was a central figure in the League for almost forty years. She first met Mrs Bagot Stack in 1931 when the League hired the hall of a ballet school for which Deidre played. She accompanied that first class and so began the association which lasted for the rest of her life. Deidre credited her own inspiration and enthusiasm for the work of the League from Mary herself, and helped to ensure her work continued after her death. Prunella describes her:

'as a woman of exceptional talent, musical knowledge and unsparing effort which were potent forces in the League's spectacular growth and success. At this time her work covered many fields: accompanying classes in the Training School for Teachers and evening League classes; arranging the music and playing at the large National Displays, held then every year at Olympia and Wembley Stadium; travelling throughout the country to play for the openings of League Centres and demonstrations; travelling abroad with a team of teachers to Sweden for the Lingiad in Stockholm in 1939 and to Germany for a Physical Education Congress in 1938; playing for beach classes during the summer holiday months; and playing on every conceivable type of piano in halls up and down the country all the year round. She never failed nor missed one day's work through illness or absence. What a wonderful friend, someone who could be utterly depended upon under any circumstance.

When the war came Deidre joined first ENSA and then the American Red Cross. She had been married in 1938 and her first home was destroyed in the 1940 blitz. They lost everything, and yet she still travelled up and down the country to give concerts to the troops and in hospitals. One of Deidre's favourite tunes which I remember her playing, is 'There's no business like show business'. After the war Deirdre helped with the rebuilding of the League. At the same time she continued with her recitals and was also much occupied with work for the BBC arranging accompaniments and coaching artists. In spite of this flowering of her talent she never failed to give the League work pride of place.'

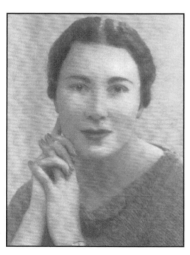

Deidre Welsh

With Madge Gillings, Deidre composed 'Marching Feet' the League song, and also wrote a considerable repertoire of other music, including the accompaniment to the 'Lingiad'. In 1933 a gramophone record was made of all the most important exercise sequences with music played and composed by Deidre herself with Madge Gillings. Deidre played at all the major events and became the League's Musical Director. Peggy St Lo wrote about her:

'There has never been a time when I haven't needed her advice and help on the musical side. We worked together so closely and she always knew what I wanted and always came up with exactly the right piece of music for me to use. At times when Joan and I became a little too ambitious regarding the musical side of a show, Deirdre would explain the difficulties involved and suggest something else – she was always right. Deidre was a tremendous 'personality' always perfectly groomed, her poise magnificent and her savoir faire the envy of us all. Underneath all the glamour was a woman with a wonderful sense of humour and fun. She had a sympathy and understanding, great integrity and a deep love and devotion for the League.'

Deidre also accompanied Prunella on many of her talks to help with the demonstrations designed to recruit new members and help set up new Centres both in the UK and abroad. At one of these, the 1932 opening of the first centre in Scotland, in Glasgow, things did not go as smoothly as planned. Part way through the Display all the lights fused and the hall was plunged into darkness. Deidre immediately decided to entertain the audience with a selection of Scottish songs which she played in the dark, as the audience sang along. As soon as the lights came on again the Display was restarted. She continued to teach at the Training School and Teacher's Refresher Courses until her retirement in 1966.

SEVENTY YEARS AT THE PIANO

There are a great number of pianists who have given decades of their lives to supporting and enlivening League classes all over the world. They are too numerous to credit individually but among them is one League pianist who has played an important role in the League for most of her life. She typifies the dedicated way in which so many have contributed to the League. Barbara Furniss has played for nearly every National display since the war and been the pianist on four Training Courses. Her composition 'Health and Beauty Parade' was the finale of the 1980 Golden Jubilee celebration. Manifesting the skills of a true improvisational pianist, Barbara began playing for the League in 1936, in London, when she was seventeen. She described her audition:

> 'Diana Ware now Kropinska was the person who gave me my very first interview and audition. Immediately after this she asked me to go and play for a teacher running a class locally. Two days later I got a letter from Madge Gillings, who was then the head pianist, saying would I please come back for another audition. Straight after that she asked me to play for the League the following week. One shilling and sixpence an hour they paid me, and I paid all my own travel. That was just before the war when I did not have another job. At that time Deidre was her assistant. They later became joint heads. Madge was a little more classical than Deidre but they were both excellent pianists. Deidre could play anything and composed many pieces. When Madge left I was asked to accompany Deidre at the Albert Hall displays. She would produce the programme and I would hear her play and then I would accompany her on the second piano.'

Now aged eighty six and semi-retired in Shropshire, Barbara spoke affectionately of her time with the League. She has a very unusual gift; she does not read music, but when she hears music she can play it. Music has always been central to her life and as she says, she is never happier than when playing. The requirements of the League, for a pianist with spontaneity and an ability to improvise, suited Barbara ideally. As she said:

'From an improvisation point of view I could fit the bill. If it was songs from the shows, I could hear the music, then my left hand would find the right notes and I could play anything. My mother and father were musical, so the mere fact that I can improvise and sit down and play for hours without looking at a note is just one of those fortunate gifts, that I have been given.

During the war I was managing a cinema in London. This was the only form of entertainment available. If I was asked if I could play somewhere then I would endeavour to do so. I would change my day off with my assistant. In the 1950's I went to South Wales with my husband and there I played for Mary Bell. If you were a teacher in those days you did not choose where you were going to teach, you were sent. Betty Urquhart had been sent from Scotland to South Wales and she asked if I could possibly play for her so I did. That started off a beautiful friendship.

When I returned to the Midlands, Betty came with me. I carried on playing regularly for the League at the Albert Hall until I was well into my sixties. I still play locally. With the League I went where I could to fit in with my lifestyle and I was belting up and down the country all the time. My husband was very patient with me. There wasn't anyone else who could take on things like the Albert Hall. I had worked with Deidre as we needed two pianists. Over time we brought the music a little bit more up to date. We also made a record of our music. Eventually the music had to be taped, as it became more difficult to find suitable pianists.'

Barbara remembered many times when she had travelled around England playing for the League. The time she went up to Blackpool with Prunella and they found that the piano for the Display had no pedals. Barbara had no choice but to carry on, although she did say there was a lot of comment on her 'poor performance'! One trip with Mary Bell, to Butlin's out of season was nearly a disaster when they were taken to the hall and not only was it freezing cold but they found that someone had removed the keyboard from the piano. Fortunately there was a second piano in another hall. Just two of the many trials and tribulations of being a mobile pianist.

It is impossible with the written word to give a sense of the role of the piano in League classes but Barbara explained to me the appeal of the piano, and why despite her age, she continues to play for the League:

'You can live with the movement, you take the music with the movement, you are not just sitting there playing or looking at a sheet of music. You are with them on the floor; or at least I find that I am. In fact one of the girls only last night at Wolverhampton noticed that I had put in extra bars to a piece as the teacher modified the exercise. In fact most of the time I can adapt what I am playing without the members or the teacher being aware of it. You cannot suddenly stop if they are trying to do something. I have loved every minute of it, and I still do.

I only play once a week now. Sometimes I feel it is a long way to go, but I get in my car and do it. And the welcome that I get, playing there, I come out reborn. So it's doing something for me too. I've done all the exercises and I have even performed in an item at the Albert Hall when they were short of performers.'

Barbara also gave an insight into the work that lies behind the major displays:

'When you are practicing for the Albert Hall then the music must be set rather than improvised. There can be up to twenty items and everything had to be set, and then taped. The pianists at the performance would then use the tapes to practice to. They used quite a lot of the minor classics. For routine exercises either Deidre or I would sort out what music we were going to use and later it would be my role to sort out the music for each item and discuss it with the teacher who was in charge of that item. The music would be circulated, so people could practice in smaller groups, and then everyone would come together for the bigger rehearsals, so that they got used to listening to the piano or tape. The teacher for each item has to have an idea of what she wants without the music, she has a rhythm; once she has the rhythm then she looks for a suitable piece of music.

Lynn Wallwork, for example, would bring me down a record and say how she wanted the music changed, to suit the sequence. I would start to play it and then she asked if I could change to a tango rhythm, and so I did, then later she wanted some Blues as there were some heavier movements, and she would tape it all. So we worked it out. The music stays with me, but I can repeat something exactly the same if I listen to the tape first.

The first time I played at the Albert Hall was the first one after the war. We often had the members piped into the Hall. We would go up to London to the Steinway studios to rehearse beforehand on two pianos. One teacher at a Display, wanted a continuous tape so there was twenty five minutes of music with one rhythm, and she asked me if I would do it, so I did it and we made eight tapes each with different rhythms. What was required was music that just went on and on and they could stop it when they wanted and when it went back on, pick up where they left off. It saved them having to rewind.'

The class in Wolverhampton understand how fortunate they are in having their exercises accompanied by Barbara. She says that it is not possible to have the spontaneity in class that the piano provides when tapes have to be used, but she does feel that the use of taped music makes the task of teaching more difficult. Considerable time and skill is required by the teacher to find the music to fit the exercises.

'From a teacher training point of view at least, I would not always play exactly the same music for the same exercise in order to give them some variety. It meant that they had to think about what they were doing rather than rely on the music, to tell them where they were. The teachers that I play for in classes do not tell me what to play, they rely on me to make the music suit the exercises. That is only because of my experience. If they suddenly say, 'Can we take this a bit slower?', or 'Can we make this into a Blues?' say instead of a waltz then OK I can do it and the piece has a different feel. It is entirely up to the teacher; if they like what I am playing they do not say anything. Sadly it looks as though I am the last of the line!'

Given Barbara's long history of performing for the League, making her the Musical Director in 1973 was an official recognition of her work, and years of loyalty. She was in charge of the music for the Displays at the Albert Hall and other venues, with all the complicated rehearsal schedules to arrange.

'I was literally in charge of the shows. Tapes were beginning to come in as it was becoming more difficult to find pianists who could adapt their playing to what the League wanted. Most of them were more accustomed to reading music and when I asked them if they could improvise, many of them were unable to.'

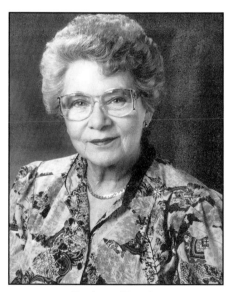

Barbara Furniss

Barbara retired as Musical Director in 1986 because by then taped music had virtually taken over, and she felt her role to be increasingly 'superfluous'. The problem in finding pianists for any event was critical and by now also finding a hall that had a piano was very difficult. However when there were major shows Barbara continued to contribute where she could, and playing for some items when asked. In 1993 she accompanied the Scottish item; which again she recorded, so she was not physically performing in the Hall. This was an item that had originally been done by Peggy and Joan and the teachers in Scotland had specifically asked that Barbara do it for them. She remembers that occasion very fondly as it reminded her of the early days. The resilience and fortitude of League members, is shared by their pianists.

Another stalwart, Dorothy Foster, at the age of ninety four, finally retired as a League pianist in 2003, having played for classes in the North West for sixty seven years.

The 'early days' are no more and the tape player is now the main source of music for teachers. In a 1966 issue of the League magazine there is a mention of the Walsall Centre holding a bring and buy sale so that they could purchase a tape recorder for the class. A small signal of an inevitable transition.

MUSIC ON THE MOVE

Displays in Hyde Park, marches and the Albert Hall meant that from the outset there was a need to find an alternative source of music to the piano. The earliest demonstrations at both venues were supported by the Band of Queen Victoria's Rifles led by Mr A. W. Selth. Mary Bagot Stack credits him with teaching the members how to synchronise their movements quickly and accurately in response to his simple system of drum beats. This came to be known as the League's 'drum beat code'. Mary observed that with his baton poised it was as if he was directing not just his band but orchestrating the co-ordinated response from the performers.

Improvisation on a wider scale was needed to ensure the right music at the wide range of different locations where the League did displays. The problems faced were many, those described by Barbara Furniss, earlier, are typical of the obstacles and handicaps that every League Pianist has had to over come in her time. There are some unusual moments from displays and some memorable moments for individuals. Fiona Gillanders related an incident at a local display:

> 'We had a show in the park and we had no tapes, but we had a pianist called Mrs Grey, I can see her now. She always wore a hat when she played the piano and she smoked. She came into the park sitting at the piano on the back of a coal lorry; so we had this view of the back of the piano and all we could see was just this hat and the cigarette smoke rising behind it!'

Coal lorries were not always available and it remains a mystery as to how so many pianos managed to find their way into the middle of fields.

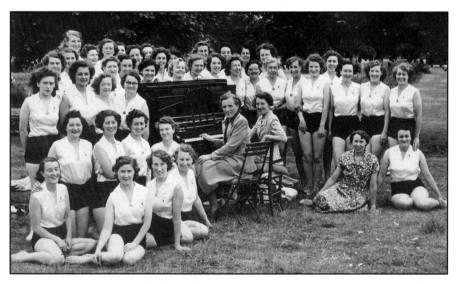

Field + piano = exercise venue

A Woburn Abbey display was held outdoors in the summer of 1968. It had rained all morning but this cleared for part of the afternoon. The two pianists, Myra Woodham and Kathleen Hilton, sat in macs and rainhoods struggling to make the pianos yield the necessary sounds! The instruments were very wet from the morning rainfall and the hammers were sticking. An unknown man in the audience came forward and put his head inside the piano and proceeded to stay there for the whole of the two performances releasing each hammer as it stuck!

League pianists are seldom called upon to play for solos dancers of quite the status of Princess Diana, but that is exactly what happened to Alice Elliott from Maidstone in June 1981. She was called to Buckingham palace to the music room where she played for forty five minutes whilst Diana danced. Quoted in the Daily Mail, a Palace spokesman said:

> 'It is designed to keep her figure in trim and her mind relaxed for that important day next month when she will marry Charles.'

It was Lady Diana's former dance teacher who knew Alice and recommended her to the Palace. Alice said afterwards that Lady Diana had not danced for some time but that she was very good and she loved it.

THE ROLE OF MUSIC TODAY

Music remains at the heart of the League, its exercises and Displays and it is an important part of any training course for teachers. As students they receive a lot of guidance in their choice of music both in relation to the tempo on the mechanics of the movements, but also on the style of the music. In Stage One they are given a CD of music with a range of tracks that are straightforward to use; simple beats that can be used with all the basic exercises. By Stage Two the students are expected to broaden the range of music they use and to explore the use of more complex rhythms and styles. They are encouraged to select music that not only suits their style of teaching but is also enjoyed by the classes they are taking. The greatest challenge to their creativity remains in the choreography of items for displays, and how the developing movements of each piece can be matched by the music.

One teacher, Liz Byrne, described how music is always at the back of her mind:

> 'The League Teacher can often be spotted browsing through the record collections in shops and libraries. The League Teacher's ear is ever aware of any music playing at any time in any place. The background beat in the dress shops could provide inspiration for next week's class. She leaves the shop, the dress forgotten, but with the warm up for her elementary class firmly fixed in the mind! The League teacher can never relax. When out for a meal is she enjoying the excellent cuisine, scenery, stimulating conversation? No! She is planning her latest workout to the inspiring music she has just heard in the background.'

Jenny Dingley explained some of the problems for a teacher in selecting the right music for her exercise class. There is a need for teachers to understand the rudiments of timing and rhythm so that when they hear a piece of music they know if it is appropriate. A teacher might hear some music that has the beat she needs but then on playing it all the way through finds that odd bars have been added at different points which mar the essential rhythm. At one time the teacher would devise the exercise and then create the music, but now it is often the case that the teacher finds the music first and then devises the exercises to go with it. All teachers try to keep the music they select modern and pleasant to listen to. There are existing recordings of piano music that has accompanied League exercises in the past but this is generally not favoured by class members, as it is deemed 'too old fashioned'. Finding suitable music can be very time consuming and expensive if you need to purchase a CD just for a single track. It seems that Shania Twain is never used because she rarely keeps to the dominant phrasing, M People on the other hand are much more reliable!

In general, though, most teachers found the use of tapes to be liberating as there was such a vast range and variety of music to choose from. In the early days not all classes could get pianists with the skills and adaptability of Deidre and Barbara. Now any teacher can have exactly the right music for the mood and tempo of the exercises or routine that she is producing. Whatever the decade, it has been the popular music of the day that has held sway.

CHAPTER 10

CONTINUITY AND CHANGE

Over the last fifty five years society has changed and the League has continued to adapt and move forward. There have been periods of growth in membership and of decline, but the League has maintained a solid membership base, due to its dedicated teachers and loyal members. The question of survival may have prompted some changes in the past but the motivation and momentum of those in leadership roles was never in doubt. There have always been financial concerns as there would be for any organisation run on such a tiny budget and reliant year to year on membership subscriptions and external grants. There are a handful of teachers in part time paid roles, but this does not realistically reflect the amount of time and effort put in by these and many others on a voluntary basis. All this has been achieved because of the continuity of the ethos and ideals of Mary Bagot Stack. It is these which ensure continued high standards of teacher training, the calibre of the exercises and the maxim that the League should be affordable to all.

Each new decade has begun with a display to celebrate a series of 'significant' birthdays. In 1950 it was held at the Empire Pool Wembley, in 1959 an early 30th birthday was celebrated at the Royal Albert Hall, while in 1970 there was a change to this pattern and a weekend Rally was held in Brighton. The next three celebrations were all held at the Albert Hall, the true home of such displays. The 1980 Golden Jubilee was a very special occasion marked by many visitors from all over the world and the awarding to Prunella of an OBE in the Queen's Birthday Honours List. Every ten years the question must rise of how to 'top that' but with a mix of traditional and new this is always achieved. At the 1990 Diamond Jubilee there were tributes to long standing teachers and members, and in 2000 there was also the welcoming in of a new millennium. Each has been central to involving and motivating members from all over the world, and each represents a new start with a renewed sense of hope.

In exploring each decade since 1950, the focus of this chapter is on the organisation of the League and some of its notable events.

THE 1950'S

From 1950 the League continued to grow with previous League Centres still being reopened and new ones being established around the UK. In 1950 there were over a thousand classes held throughout the country each week. Readjustments following the war years were still being made at all levels in the organisation. Since 1941 the League had operated as a private limited company, a form of company that had been adopted to meet wartime circumstances. By 1950 Mr McLeod, the League treasurer, suggested that this was a suitable time to change the League's constitution, to a non-profit making Association, with unlimited membership and with charity status. Prunella believed that these steps would help to ensure stability and permanence, and many well known figures in education, health and sport came forward to support the League. The League was financially stable with a capital of £1,000 donated to it by the shareholders of the former company, and one of the first actions was to develop a reserve fund from which the teacher training would be financed.

The business of the Association was managed by a Council consisting of not less than five members. In fact the Council was set up with eleven members acting in honorary capacity, and an Executive of five, who each continued in their previous duties, to guide and control the day to day affairs which affected teachers and members. The Executive comprised the Organising Secretary, the Company Secretary and three or four teachers representing different areas, who served set terms. Peggy St Lo was appointed as Organising Secretary, a position she held until 1983.

The Council decided to conduct a survey of members in 1955. The cost of distributing the questionnaire to every member was prohibitive, so a cross section of members was selected. A total of one thousand members over the age of twenty one, from six Centres, were surveyed, and eight hundred and seventy two forms were completed. The consistency between replies from each centre added to confidence levels that the responses were representative. It was discovered that 40% of members had joined within the previous year and 67% of members had joined through the recommendation of a friend, 17% from local publicity, 17% from a League demonstration and 7% from national publicity. The dominance of 'word of mouth' has been a feature of League recruitment throughout. 80% said that the main benefit they gained from attending League classes was a sense of well being and 39% mentioned social contacts as a major benefit. This percentage was higher in smaller compact areas. For over 70% of members the League was their only outlet for any form of physical recreation, and for over 80% the League was the only society to which they belonged. The information that 75% of members practiced at home between classes, is interesting, as is the fact that there were forty seven instances of both mothers and daughters attending the same class.

Prunella had spent seven years living in South Africa, but had maintained close contact with the Council, Peggy and Joan St Lo and others. In 1956 she made a very welcome return, with her two sons, to England. The following year saw a particularly successful time for the League with the opening of several new Centres in Barrow in Furness, Bridgewater, Burton-on –Trent, Chelmsford, Harlow, Hull, Lancaster, Salisbury and Swindon, and other centres were re-opened in Huddersfield, Oxford, Stoke-on-Trent, and Sunderland. By 1958 there were one hundred and thirty five Centres in Britain, with over six hundred weekly classes, and an active membership of thirty thousand. Fewer classes than at the start of the decade but overall membership was higher. Quite remarkably the cost of classes by then had only risen to just one shilling with the annual fee standing at seven shillings.

THE 1960'S

New centres continued to open, with most classes being full. Other activity was also on the increase as more centres were putting on rallies and displays or taking part in other local events. In the summer of 1961 during May, June and July, there were over thirty eight different events and demonstrations across the country. Despite all this, financial pressures were beginning to grow. At the Annual General Meeting in 1964 it was reported that there were still three factors that were putting pressure on the League's finances: the cost of the training college, subsidising the magazine and the provision of a teacher's pension. A very welcome grant had been received from the Department of Education and Science, which was designated for administrative purposes.

On a happier front, in May 1964 Prunella married Brian St Quentin Power. It was a small wedding with just family and a few close friends, but the warmest wishes were sent to her by everyone in the League, for a very happy future. The following year saw Prunella continuing her promotional visits on behalf of the League. In April fifty representatives from industry, commerce and the press attended a Conference at the Shell Centre South Bank, to discuss the idea of some form of physical training in co-operation with industry. The Conference was sponsored by the League and Prunella spoke about the framework of the League and listed the services it could offer. She gave two examples in the London area, the John Lewis Partnership and the Prudential Assurance Company Limited, where classes had been held for some time. Anne Lillis talked about how strain and tiredness was not directly related to the amount of time spent working but to the way in which work was done. It was suggested that League class would make a valuable contribution to a company's social and sports activities, especially if the classes could take place within the company itself. It was proposed that companies should be asked to participate in trials whereby they could compare outcomes for the participants, with the average employee who had not taken such a course. There is no record as to uptake. However, by the end of the 1960's League teachers were again expanding their horizons and taking League classes beyond their Centres. Classes were being taught in over sixteen schools, thirteen Further Education Day and Evening Centres, eight mental hospitals, two institutions for the handicapped, five retirement classes and many more other types of social club. Unlike the war years only three commercial organisations hosted classes, John Lewis and Co, Glenn Line Shipping and the Prudential Assurance Company.

THE 1970'S

The League Council resolved that 1970 would be 'publicity year' starting with the 40th Birthday Brighton Rally and aiming to appear frequently in the news media throughout the country. For this, the League brought in external professional assistance. Another notable occurrence that year was that is was the first time that the Council had officially discussed the possibility of changing the name of the League at the AGM. It was particularly sad that any mood of optimism for the future was to be clouded by the closure of the Bagot Stack College. The outcome of the closure was that at the 1972 AGM, the chairman was able to report a 'satisfactory surplus' on accounts. This, he told members, was due to two factors, firstly that no full time training of teachers had been carried out during 1971, and that the Department of the Environment had renewed its grant towards Headquarters administration.

Complementing the publicity drive, Prunella's book "Movement is Life" was published in 1973. It received very positive publicity which enhanced the reputation of the League. It was made into an audio tape read by Phyllis Boothroyd, and it was serialised in Woman's Weekly. Prunella also made many media appearances. She was interviewed on Woman's Hour; ATV's Women Today, Harlech TV's Women Only, Southern TV's House Party; and Scottish TV's Dateline. In addition to this there were a large number of reviews in journals and papers both in the UK and in South Africa. As one review said: 'The women of the early League are the prototypes of the figure conscious, yoga practicing, health food women of today.' Even the New Statesman and its noted contributor the sardonic Arthur Marshall, deemed the book worthy of review. His review, in his inimitable style, follows:

> 'It is not Prunella Stack's fault that the mere mention of her name conjures up, for the middle-aged, a picture of less than lissom ladies striving gamely for health and beauty to the sound of portable gramophone, straining serge and busting bloomer. These activities were, in fact, the invention of her mother, Mary Bagot Stack, suddenly inspired while at morning exercise. In no time at all, all women were leaping and hopping and breathing in all directions with Prunella doing the donkey work of organising, after her mother's untimely death. Miss Stack has known great tragedy but as one tip toes through the clichés in this likeable autobiography, cheerfulness and goodness keep breaking through and she remains the League's best advertisement.' (9.3.73)

Another new venture that year was the production of the League's first LP, i.e. long playing record. The production team had been Joan and Peggy St Lo, Betty Urquhart and Barbara Furniss.

All this publicity and effort was thrown into turmoil the following year when a number of Centres faced temporary closure due to the fuel crisis, and where they did not close attendance was greatly reduced. Publicity soon became a secondary issue, as the impact on teachers' income, became clear. An addition of five pence per subscription was made to contribute towards a 'Crisis Fund', which would enable the League to assist teachers in the future should a similar problem arise.

A longer lasting change also came about in 1974, and one that was far more controversial. Even thirty years later many members mourn this day. The Executive Committee had approved a black and white leotard for class wear only, but not for displays. All members were requested to maintain the League's standards by keeping to the black and white colour scheme. The Leotard was all in one with a white blouse top with collar and front zip, attached to 'snug fitting' black pants and was made of nylon. This break from the traditional black satin pants and white satin blouse was not well received by many long standing members. They thought that this would be the 'thin end of the wedge' and the end of the uniform. As history shows they were quite right. Leotards were, by the seventies, the garment of choice for exercise and it was a necessary decision to follow this trend, to ensure newer members preferences were taken into account. In the long term most members would probably agree that it was a small price to pay to ensure that the League was not viewed as 'outdated'.

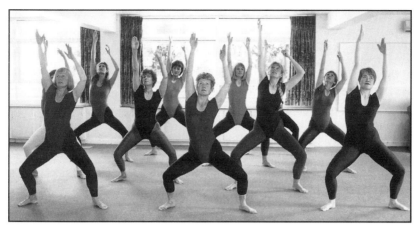

Leotards in class

In 1976 it was announced by the chairman Mr Denis Richards at the AGM, that there was a very welcome surplus of £7,000 on the main account, £4,000 of which had been due to the great success of the Albert Hall show. This was put in reserve for any future deficits. Further good news was received that Prunella had been awarded the Jubilee Medal in recognition of the work of the League. There was also a welcome increase in League membership. However by 1977 there was a £3,000 deficit and it was proposed to tackle this by expanding the membership. The aim was to re-achieve a membership of thirty thousand by 1980. In the financial year ending September 1978 there were twenty eight thousand members and the good news was that there was a surplus on the account, but the bad news was that it was only £55!

The decade ended with a return to another hot chestnut, the renaming of the League. To be absolutely correct, the proposal was for the League to adopt a new 'working title', whilst constitutionally remaining the 'Women's League of Health and Beauty'. In 1979 the AGM again debated this issue with the majority favouring the dropping of the word 'Women's' from the title. This was to be put to a vote of the membership. Prunella was in favour of the name change as she recognised that many saw the name as too long and too old fashioned.

THE 1980'S

The outcome of the vote on the adoption of a new name, was that 44% of the Associate membership voted for removing the word 'Women's', 15% favoured 'Health and Beauty Movement', whilst 41% felt that no change was desirable. The number of Associate members was two thousand and eighty nine. Any ordinary member could become and Associate by the payment of an additional subscription fee. This gave them the right to vote on important issues such as this. However when the next meeting was held in March 1981, and the issue was put to the vote again, it was defeated. There would be no change at this time. During 1980 membership dropped by a thousand.

The AGM in 1981 reduced the size of the Council from twenty five to just twelve. This was to reflect the change in the role of the Council as Mr Denis Richards explained:

'Conditions have changed over the thirty years of the life of the Association and from being a rather grand and ornamental body which met once a year, the Council was now a Board which met frequently and had various sub-committees, to conduct the complex workings of a large organisation.'

This resolution was passed by a large majority. The first year of the Eighties was good financially, helped by the success of the Golden Jubilee show and the continuation of the Sports Council Grant which was a 'significant help'.

Another significant event occurred in 1982: it was the centenary of Mary Bagot Stack's birth. Contributions were sought for the Bagot Stack Centenary Fund to provide Stoke Mandeville Hospital with a lasting memorial of her life and work. In April a Bagot Stack Centenary Fund celebration took place in London and on the first day a cheque for £3,000 was presented to the Sports Centre at Stoke Mandeville. On the second day, as Prunella noted, 'a cheque of truly staggering proportions' for £24,180 was presented to Dr H Frankel from Stoke Mandeville, for the New Building Fund. A plaque commemorating the life and work of Mrs Stack was placed in the new building when it was completed, in 1985.

In 1982 Prunella was made President designate of the League. It required an Extraordinary General Meeting in 1983 to enable the new appointment of a President to be made. A by now routine item at the AGM that followed was the proposal to change the name to 'Health and Beauty Movement' but it was again defeated. In 1984 Peggy St Lo retired from her administrative role and she was elected onto the Council. She and Joan were made Vice-Presidents of the League in honour of all their work and support.

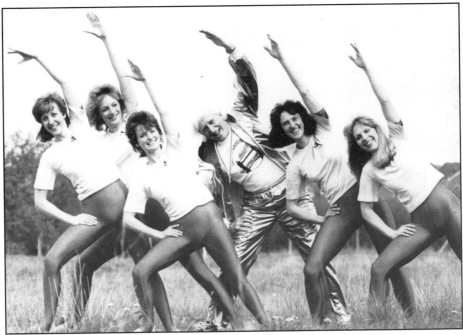

The League at Stoke Mandeville Hospital with Jimmy Saville

The next year saw a number of events. Many Centres celebrated their Golden Jubilees, as 1935 was the year that saw the opening of the largest number of centres in any one year. The League's new Press Officer gained valuable publicity on TV and a new record and video made by the League, were selling well. The video had been screened at the Healthier Living Exhibition at Earl's Court. Called 'Do It In Style' it showed exercises with music chosen from recent hits and with a voice over by Lucy Martin. That same year there was a small deficit on the accounts and there had been a small decline in membership. The AGM called for the recruitment of more teachers as existing teachers were now holding fewer classes.

At a Sports Council Grants panel meeting in 1986, the League was urged to shorten and update its name. The tide turned and the working title of 'Health and Beauty Exercise' was adopted. The Sports Council also wanted to see more involvement of teenagers, school leavers, those up to twenty five and young mothers with children. The Council formed a subcommittee and a plan was developed to attract younger members by having classes especially for them. This new venture was called STYLE, Slimming, Toning, Youthful, Lively Exercise. Brightly coloured leotards were slowly appearing in classes by now, so with the accompaniment of pop music the new classes were launched.

There were further administrative changes that year with the appointment of Regional Officers being made official, whereas up until then they had been voluntary. They were to receive a yearly fee and were asked to spend more time taking over the ever expanding role previously taken by the National Development Officer. This included seeking regional publicity and sponsorship and ensuring that there was an annual regional rally, as well as responding to the Sports Councils requests for more classes for the young, new mothers, and ethnic groups.

In 1986 a project was initiated in the USA to symbolise the achievement of women in Western Civilisation. Two Southgate League members Joan Brooks and Hilda Taylor produced a quilt in honour of the Women's League of Health and Beauty. The 'Honour Quilt' was worked in black and white satin with the name of the founder, Mrs Bagot Stack, and that of Prunella, in filled chain stitch. The motto 'Movement is Life' was couched in continuous white thread on the black panel. This was remarkable piece of work which was put on show in the UK and was then sent to the US to join seven hundred 'Honour Quilts' from all over the world. There was no mention of its final destination.

In 1987 the League mourned the death of Joan St Lo. Her life and long list of achievements was celebrated at a memorial service held for her in London that Autumn.

By the late Eighties there were increasing numbers of members wearing leotards of different designs in classes and the League introduced their own brand of leotards in a range of designs and colours, which had two white 'V' inserts, and the Leap logo. The demise of the black and white themed clothing was now official.

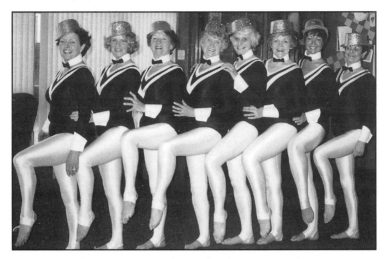

The new League leotard - plus accessories!

As the legal responsibilities of Council as Charity Governors grew, in 1989 a member of the Council was appointed to attend the Executive Committee meetings which were held approximately every six weeks. In this way all sections of management and the teachers and members could be in close communication. The role of the Executive Committee was explained:

> 'The Executive Committee meets about eight times a year and its role is to assist the League Secretary in the day to day running of the organisation. The main responsibility is to support and advise teachers in the running of their classes. We also advise and receive reports from the Regional Development Officers and Liaison Officer, deal with queries from outside the League and enact Council recommendations.'

As the responsibilities of the chair of the Executive Committee increased, it was agreed to create an additional post of Liaison Officer. Initially this role was combined with that of chair and was taken by Rosemary Barber.

THE 1990's

Major birthday celebrations catch the eye of the press, and following the 1990 Diamond Jubilee Week, the YOU magazine of the Mail on Sunday wrote:

> 'Twenty thousand ladies leaping. Eat your heart out Jane Fonda; the Women's League of Health and Beauty threw away their corsets before you were even born. And in the League's Diamond Jubilee year great grandmothers at the peak of fitness still draw glances.'

Building on the publicity potential, Prunella made many radio and television appearances that year, and articles were written about the League in several leading magazines, including Good Housekeeping, Saga, Weight Watchers, and Bella.

An Incentive Scheme Trophy was awarded to the Region with the highest percentage increase in membership. For 1990/1 it was won by the Scottish Western Region and the following year by the Scottish Eastern region. In the following year thirty two new classes were set up and there was an increase in membership. A survey among teachers showed that there were one hundred and ninety seven active teachers taking six hundred and twenty six separate weekly classes across the UK. By September 1993 there were over three hundred Centres in the UK with more than twenty thousand members, and the Executive Committee were monitoring the progress of the thirty three new centres which had opened in 1992, while fourteen more were due to start in the Autumn of 1993. The Health and Beauty Exercise financial support scheme was introduced as a valuable backup to new classes, as it guaranteed that teachers did not lose money in the first year of their classes and it assisted with advertising costs. Unfortunately that year the Sports Council reduced its grant to the League.

The move of head office to Chertsey Surrey in 1994 accompanied a realignment of roles, with the administration being taken over by a number of teachers: Val Augustine became Administration Officer, Rosemary Barber Internal Liaison, Margaret Peggie External Liaison, and Lucy Martin Training Officer.

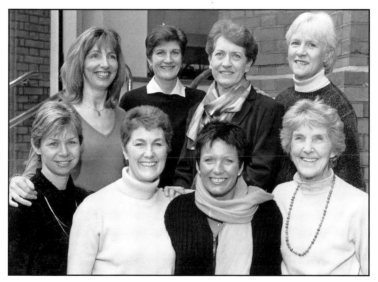

Council members and teachers: top l-r Jill Shipton, Margaret McAllister, Rosemary Barber, Lucy Martin, bottom l-r Julia Durbin, Margaret Peggie, Lyn Hicks, with President Prunella Stack

With regards to the name of the League, 1995 saw a return to an earlier debate, as the AGM again discussed an alternative to 'Health and Beauty Exercise'. This arose primarily because it was reported by teachers that many prospective members were asking when the 'make-up' lessons took place! The inclusion of the word 'Beauty' was also felt by many members to deter others from joining. Pat Rowlandson threw the challenge out to members to see what suggestions they might have. The response was overwhelming. The majority asked for the word 'League' to be reinstated. Others pointed out that changing the name again would make for confusion and loss of identity. However at this stage, there was to be no change.

In 1995 Margaret McAllister coined the name MANFIT for a class she was dragooned into running for a group of – to quote the men themselves – 'unfit and largely middle aged men'. One of their number, David White said:

'It all came about because I had seen a most interesting TV documentary in the USA made by some leading orthopaedic surgeons on the incidence of back problems. Their studies had led them to conclude that 2% of sufferers needed surgery while 98% needed regular exercise. I met Margaret and spent some time trying to persuade her to run one of her classes for a bunch of men. She finally said that if I could round up ten or more willing victims she would take us on. We started with fifteen but within six months it had grown to thirty three. For the sake of our egos Margaret allowed us to delete 'Women' and 'Beauty' from the standard membership form which made us feel much better. We are approaching the end of our first year slimmer and very considerably more flexible.'

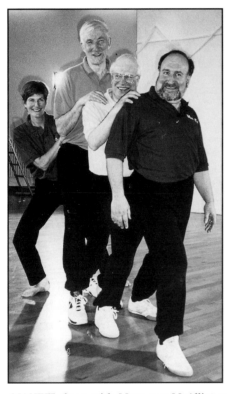

MANFIT class with Margaret McAllister.

In 1996 a survey sent to three hundred and fifty members who did not renew their membership found only ten had been dissatisfied with classes. Many were only temporarily absent whilst some had increased business pressures and others had succumbed to the ageing factor. This evidence was reassuring as it was predominantly circumstances beyond the League's control that resulted in this decline in membership and that the standard of classes remained as high as ever.

In 1997 Prunella and Margaret Peggie received an invitation to represent the League at a reception at Buckingham Palace by the Central Council of Physical Recreation (CCPR). This was held to honour the sporting life of the nation. The Queen, Prince Philip, Princess Anne, and Princes Andrew and Edward were present, with seven hundred guests. As a member of the CCPR Executive, Margaret Peggie joined the retinue that followed Prince Philip and the General Secretary. As she wrote at the time:

'It was wonderful to be inside the palace and to view all those amazingly ornate rooms which are so immaculately kept. I spoke or was spoken to by Prince Philip, Prince Andrew, Prince Edward and the Duke of Gloucester. I suppose it is rather disrespectful to say that one of the highlights was driving my car through the gates of the palace, then sweeping (oh yes I swept) through one of the arches where the sentry guards stand in the inner courtyard where, would you believe it, I drove tremblingly under the canopy to the front door where I deposited CCPR passengers. From there I was directed to park alongside the canopy outside the royal front door.'

The League produced two more videos, 'Inside-Out' and 'ManFit' in 1998 and became hooked up to the internet with an e-mail address and plans to develop a web page. The Executive Committee produced its first Equal Opportunities Policy. It had always practiced equal opportunities but a written policy was deemed appropriate as this was increasingly being required by external bodies.

The major milestone of the coming millennium and the League's 70th birthday, led the Council to look closely at what they were doing and what they might do in the future. At that time Prunella wrote of the need to look outwards, and to reach the many potential members who would join if only they knew of the League. The Chairman of the Executive Committee wrote of the increasingly tough time teachers were facing having to compete with the plethora of alternative, fashionable and commercial classes. An incentive scheme for members was introduced for those who introduced the most new members to their class. Research carried out by the League showed that teachers and existing members wholeheartedly believed in the value of the Bagot Stack system and that it continued to fulfil a very important need.

The Council had decided that there was need for further change and they brought in a full time manager from outside, Joyce Turton, to replace the part time roles of different teachers. The choice of manager was made on the basis that her main skills were in marketing. The Executive Committee was renamed the Liaison Committee. One of the new manager's key decisions was to recruit a PR consultant to promote the League. Other things did not change as debate about the working name for the League continued. 'Health and Beauty Exercise' was seen as a hindrance when advertising classes and ideas for a new name were still being sought. Prompted by Joyce, this finally became a reality in 1999 when the name 'The Fitness League' was selected and, by popular demand, the 'Leap' logo was reinstated on the cover of the magazine.

THE NEW MILLENNIUM

Barely a year after the creation of the Liaison Committee in lieu of the Executive Committee, it was disbanded. It was also decided to cease the post of Liaison Officer. This marked a very significant change away from the integrated form of management established to that date. Management control had been centralised into a single role and well established links between the teachers and head office were broken. This would inevitably have an impact upon the quality of internal communications. The informal networks among teachers, especially those who had been closely involved with League management in the past, did continue and carried a greater weight of responsibility for the continuing co-ordination of affairs than would usually be warranted.

The year 2000 was also memorable because the League went global via the world wide web. This was seen as the perfect way to keep in close touch with others all over the world twenty four hours a day, and became the easiest way for anybody to find information about the League, the classes or to have discussions or to send messages. It could not however replace other structures when it came to teacher liaison as many teachers did not have access to the internet.

A new venture that year was to sell a range of souvenirs marking the 70th birthday celebrations. These were classic in design from a silver plated handbag mirror, to Dartington Glass rose bowls and bud vase, to the practical ball point pen and tea towel, each bearing the League's logo. No competition, though, for the teddy bear wearing a League sweatshirt. The most delightful and lasting gift was the Prunella Stack rose which would give pleasure to many, for decades to come.

2001 began with the very sad news of the death of Peggy St Lo. The tributes flooded in and a Thanksgiving service was held for her at Bloomsbury Baptist Church in London. The following year an inscribed bench in memory of the St Lo sisters was placed in Hyde Park.

Following on from the management shake up of the previous year, in 2001 it was decided to dispense with the full time paid role of manager. This had been an interesting and, now acknowledged, expensive experiment. Although it had not been intended as an experiment it was fortunate that it was one from which the Council learnt many lessons. It may be politically expedient to respond to suggestions that the League needed to 'modernise' but exactly what this means for one organisation is seldom the same as for others.

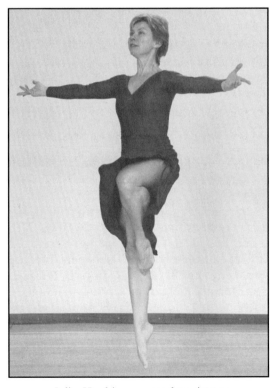

Julia Hopkins - a modern image

The Council appointed a new Chairman in 2003, Peter Hobden, who as one of that famous breed, a 'League Husband', brought with him valuable familiarity with the ethos and workings of the organisation, to which he added his business expertise. As the League in the UK focused on re-establishing its management and administrative systems, the Leagues' in New Zealand and South Africa decided to follow the UK in adopting the new name and logo and in formally affiliating themselves with the UK organisation. The League network could only be strengthened by such moves.

There were increasing concerns about the future of the grants which the League received from the Sports Council, and at their suggestion an informal partnership was created between The Fitness League, the Keep Fit Association, Medau, Margaret Morris Movement and the English Folk Dance Society. This was formalised in 2004 with the formation of an independent association called the Exercise, Movement and Dance Partnership. This was very timely as the Sport England grant was due to run out in March 2005, and in the future they would only liaise with the new Association. This Partnership remains largely informal until such time as the various ways these different groups might co-operate and work together can be established.

The year 2004 is best remembered as Prunella's 90th birthday. She was presented with a book of 'memories' compiled by Lynn Berry on behalf of the Teacher's Association, at a party organised by the teachers in Torquay. This contained each teacher's memories of Prunella over the lifetime of the League. Prunella may no longer work full time with the League but she continues to give it her support and visits Centres and Displays to promote the League whenever she can. Her wisdom and experience remains a valuable asset to the Council.

The present day sees preparations for the 2005 seventy fifth birthday celebrations at the Albert Hall in full swing. The aim is to make it the biggest yet and a suitable fanfare to welcome in the next seventy five years for the League.

CHAPTER 11

JOINING FOR LIFE

Why do members, once they have joined, tend to remain for life? The comments made by new members in 2005 can be remarkably similar to those who have been members for over fifty years. Their thoughts and feelings about the League echo those of members who wrote to the magazine in the early years. The two most familiar words used are 'fun' and 'friendship'.

WHAT MEMBERS SAY

In 1992 there was a survey of League members with almost seven thousand responses. When asked about what they liked about League classes, almost all mentioned the type of exercise and the quality of the teaching. Over half mentioned the atmosphere and the social aspect. The majority had heard about the League because a friend or relative was a member. Four out of ten had been a member for more than ten years, and all thought that it was excellent value when compared with health club or gym membership. More recently, an increasing number of day time classes have been opening, but two thirds of members attended classes in the evening.

Recent interviews have been held with twenty members across the country who had joined the League between three and sixty eight years ago. When they were asked about why they joined, it was either because a friend or relative was a member or they had it recommended to them by a friend or acquaintance. Here are just a few of the responses:

> 'We joined in 2002, four of us aged between fifty two and fifty seven. We were introduced by a friend; we all go down the gym to swim, and she was so enthusiastic that you couldn't help but say you'd give it a go. Since we have been going we have never stopped laughing. The difference between this class and a gym is that here you are part of a family, you are made welcome and people are concerned if you are not there. At a gym nobody asks or cares if you go every week.'

> 'I was a new mum; it was in 1993, and a woman I met at ante natal classes told me about it, and I felt that I wanted to do something for me. I attended first class and it was a wonderful, friendly and lively class with plenty of dance and movement that I felt comfortable with. I was made to feel very welcome and I felt really happy when I was there, not only was the class doing something for me physically but mentally it was the prop I needed.'

> 'It was 1986 when I joined, I was eighteen. I knew about it from friends who recommended it as I had a back problem.'

> 'I joined Junior Classes in 1975 when I was eight, and have been a

member ever since.'

'I was looking for something to do. I had had my family and I was not working then, that would be 1974. My neighbour told me about it. When you first go you are mesmerised, you think I could never do this, but very soon, you are! The one thing that struck me was the teacher, she was so confident.'

Several of the members and teachers who joined at a young age were introduced to the League because their mothers were members. Many have stayed in the League ever since. Fiona Gillanders and her mother Jean Yuill are typical of these. As Fiona said:

'I joined when I was twenty months old in 1949. My mother was a League teacher and so I was actually in the League before I was born. I appeared as a lump at many shows and on many platforms. I performed in shows at the age of two.'

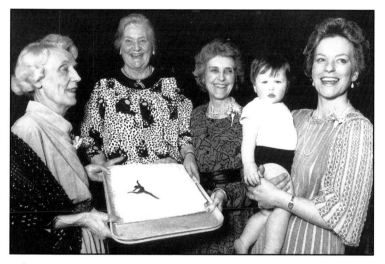

l-r Peggy St Lo, Jean Yuill, Prunella Stack, Mhairi with mother
Fiona Gillanders, celebrating Jean's 50 years of teaching.

Members who have been in the League over forty years tell very similar stories;

'I joined the Keep Fit Association to start with. My friend and I went along. The teacher started late finished early, with a long break. Then a friend told me about the Women's League of Health and Beauty, and I thought what on earth is that? It sounds awful but she persuaded us to come. I think that was 1960. From the very first week I was hooked. The teacher was brilliant, she explained everything so you knew exactly what you were doing and why.'

'I joined in 1958, my aunt held classes and I had been to see a few demonstrations so I tried it and was hooked.'

'I went along to a fete, it was 1953, and the League were doing a ribbon dance that a friend was in and I was amazed, it was wonderful, so when I got home I wrote to the local organiser, I went along to a class and I was hooked straight away.'

'At school I was gymnastics crazy and afterwards I wanted to carry on. I first went to keep fit and then changed to the League in 1954 after my children were born as people at work were talking about it. The first time I went I was so impressed, there were about sixty people there. I liked the style and the teaching impressed me.'

'I joined in 1947. My sister went to classes in her factory during the war and after that class disbanded she gave me her pants and blouse and that was when Kathleen Ward was opening a class in Hay Mills Birmingham. I had been a dancer, and I was pleased to be able to do something that involved movement. I had a baby and my husband looked after her when I went to class. I had had an operation to have part of my lung removed and my husband wanted me to go the League as it would help with my breathing.'

'I joined the League in 1937 when I was fourteen. It's been my life.'

Only one of those interviewed had remained single, and of those that married several stressed how important the support and help of their husbands and families had been when they became involved with displays, weekends away and additional classes. In the early days there had been many members who stopped going to classes when they married. Among those interviewed only one had a husband who disapproved and another member said that it was her sister who was most critical of her for leaving her husband and children at weekends. Looking back, many had not seen themselves as 'emancipated' but all of them had been determined to continue with classes and made whatever domestic arrangement were necessary. If husbands were not available then mothers or friends would be asked to help.

By contrast there were far more references to that special breed of male, the 'League Husband'. Their role may have been predominantly child minding or getting their own meals, but a few stalwarts have given much more to the League from behind the scenes. Fiona Gillanders recalls her father's support for her mother Jean Yuill, in his role of general assistant, which involved taxi driving, time keeping in practice sessions, keeping open house and catering for different groups, as well as being an excellent stage manager at Displays. The lucky few have accompanied their wives on exotic trips to far off places, and an even smaller number have actually joined MANFIT League classes themselves!

Describing the classes, there were many insights into why so many members end up staying in the League for life. As one member so clearly put it:

'It does not matter what shape or size you are, there's no competition. You only do what you feel comfortable doing you never force yourself. When you do sequences you do not have to be perfect but you try to be; it looks really good. It is very important to make time for yourself. It helps you stress wise. It is totally relaxing but your brain has to work as well, you have got to think about movement and breathing, so you are very focused. I once tried a rowing machine and on that you do not have to think at all and it was so boring. At class you never get bored, the two hours goes so quickly, the slightest movement is toning you up. And everyone chats a lot, even when you are supposed to be exercising! '

Like many others, that member expressed great regret that she had not joined many years earlier. There was also a strong feeling that many more people would enjoy the classes and get benefit if only they knew about them. Although several members also attended the local gym this was only when there were no large membership fees, and it was mainly to enjoy facilities such as the sauna, swimming pool and café, and not the classes on offer.

What all the members interviewed shared was a continuing enthusiasm. All spoke at length about the fun they had had through League events and the friends they had made. Weekends away with the League whether as a 'holiday' or practice session, always afforded sufficient free time for them to 'let their hair down'; whether it was getting out of the lift on the wrong floor, very late at night, dressed in your pyjamas, empty bottle and glass of wine in hand, looking for your room, or trying to get to the pub a few miles from Lilleshall and accepting a lift from fellow residents, who just happened to be rugby players. Rest assured, rooms were eventually found and the pub goers had a very good friend who crept downstairs in the middle of the night to unlock the main doors to let them back in!

From such strong friendships comes support in hard times. Several mentioned how League friends had helped when they had suffered illness or bereavement. Others said that it was the one place they knew they could go where they would get understanding and not excessive fuss. Peggy Bold, a member for fifty eight years, recounted how grateful she was for what the League had done for her:

> 'I think the League was my saviour when my husband was ill, he was ill for nearly ten years. I'd be at the hospital all day, but I would still go straight on to the League, after a very stressful day, I would go to the League and relax and do my exercises. I'd then go back home feeling satisfied. The League helped me to keep going, helped me cope with the difficulties and made me able to face another day.'

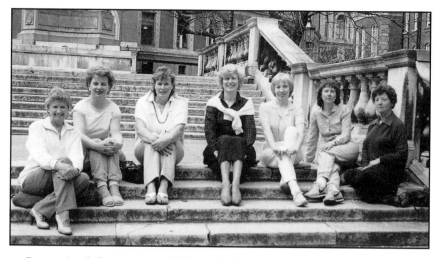

Peggy (on left) on steps of Albert Hall with other Midland members in 2000. Over 250 membership years between them!

Fitness and Well Being

Another very common theme amongst those interviewed and in magazine articles, was the great health benefits that being League members had brought. As Rosemary Barber noted:

> 'We have had some members for very many years and sometimes when you see them you are astonished at how old they are. I know of one active member who is ninety two and I have a member of eighty six who has been in the League since 1947. Until five years ago she could still do the splits, and physically she looks twenty years younger. Mentally she is very alert and it is that that makes you think – there is something in this!'

All members acknowledged that their mobility and suppleness was greater since they joined the League. Most had stories about illness or injury and their own recoveries that had surprised their doctors:

> 'I broke my leg and my first thought was 'Oh my, I am not going to be able to do Health and Beauty any more.' It was a bad break and I needed to have a plate fitted, but when it mended I was told I did not need physiotherapy as I was so supple.'

> · 'I proved the doctors and physiotherapists wrong when they told me that I would not regain full movement in my arm after a rotor cup repair. I was in my seventies but I persevered with my League exercises and four years later I am one hundred per cent fit again.'

A very great number of earlier examples and quite amazing stories can be found in the League magazine. To take but a few examples: in 1964 Winifred Entwhistle who had been a nurse and had always suffered from back pains, had a fall, and her back condition worsened:

> 'Then followed visit after visit to doctors' surgeries, specialists, wearing an appallingly restrictive corset and months of treatment at the hospital. After two years my condition had become chronic. I spent long hours on the bed, sitting upright in a chair and all cooking sitting on a stool. After that I tried the unorthodox and paid repeated visits to an osteopath. When he assured me he could do no more and suggested the wearing of another type of corset, I decided to abandon treatment and carried on living the life of a woman of advanced years, walking with a stick and unable to climb stairs at the age of 48! A year later I was persuaded to visit a newly opened clinic of a physiotherapist. After my first visit I felt I had found someone who understood and could help me. I went twice a week for four months, ending each day with strengthening exercises. The physiotherapist suggested that I join the League as he said its exercises followed very closely those he had given me. By then I had abandoned my stick, but I felt very strange and wobbly at the first evening. The teacher was most kind and helpful, telling me in advance of certain movements that I should sit out. It was not many months before I was able to go through the whole elementary class and the following year took part in an exhibition class. I have never looked back, I now feel more normal, younger and happier than I have done for six years.'

This may read like a one off testimonial for an advert but is typical of the stories told by members at classes all over the country. The League magazine continues to be full of such stories like that of Jill Dixon who wears metal callipers on her legs, having a rare neurological condition similar to Cerebral Palsy. Having seen many specialists and received regular physiotherapy nothing helped her condition. Her neurologist suggested she did exercise but after ten years Jill had gained some benefit from them but still could not lift her legs. A new teacher in her League class, Kathryn Gluyas, spent nine months working with Jill, gradually building up movements that had previously been impossible. Now Jill can lift her knee and walking is much easier as are stairs and getting in and out of cars. Most weeks Jill manages to do most of the class exercises, and recently she rode a bike for the first time since childhood. Jill believes that the League has changed her life although it is also clear that such huge improvements have a lot to do with her own determination and perseverance.

In September 1975 League teacher Georgina Heyhoe was involved in a road accident and fractured the second and third Cervical Vertebrae of her neck and as she said, she was lucky to be alive as these are the bones which break when anyone is hanged! After being transferred to Stoke Mandeville Spinal Unit, some muscle tone was recovered, and Georgina struggled to do exercises to move her feet and toes. She was then so grateful for the benefit that years of League exercises had done for her. The doctors expected her to recover sufficiently to walk with the help of aids, but because she was fit and worked hard on her exercises she had a far greater range of movement and more strength than the doctors could ever have anticipated. Her walking without aids improved and by September 1976 just one year later, she was back teaching her class.

Medical research on identical twins is of great value because any differences between the twins in old age can more confidently be associated with lifestyle. An article in the League magazine in 2000, related the case of Hilda Lewis and her identical twin Sheila. Then sixty three, they were invited to take part in the Twin Research Unit's programme at St Thomas' Hospital in London. The unit is researching the role of genetic versus environmental factors in the development of diseases and conditions related to old age. Hilda had been a member of the League for thirty six years whilst her sister had not. Hilda's bone density was much greater than that of her sister, and while Hilda remained healthy and had never broken any bones, Sheila suffered from Rheumatoid Arthritis and had had operations on the joints of her toes and had fractured her leg on two occasions. The research is still ongoing, but the results to date strongly suggest that Hilda's membership of the League has played a significant role. There are thousands more stories out there. The League magazine editor Caroline Quigley says that she is sent so many that she cannot possibly print them all.

Being in the League gives women more 'life' in so many ways, and with many areas having junior classes it is possible to be a League member for the whole of one's life. Junior League classes have been available from the very start, and classes that are specially tailored for teenagers have been introduced more recently under the acronym STYLE. When members continue going to classes into old age, they remain sufficiently supple to continue in ordinary classes. There are particular issues when the elderly begin exercising for the first time, and this need has led to the creation of EXTEND which is an offshoot of the League designed for those with limited mobility.

JUNIOR LEAGUE

The very first classes held by Mary Bagot Stack in the 1920's were for children. However it was not until 1936 that the Junior League was officially established and there were soon two thousand eight hundred members with over ninety classes each week. Many of today's members and teachers first joined as children, and there has been a strong tradition of daughters following their mothers into the League. The popularity of junior classes has varied over time and between different areas, but they have become established not only all over the UK but in other countries as well.

The League's form of physical education has been adapted to benefit under fives, as well as children as they grow to adulthood. The main 'problem' for such classes is that young grow up and so there is a need for continuous recruitment. An issue with school age children is that they are not always home from school in time for early evening classes. If numbers are too small in a class, then it may be difficult to find a suitably priced hall. As with adults, some young pupils with posture problems and other more serious conditions are sent to League classes by doctors.

Each class is carefully planned with regard to the children's physiological and psychological needs. Classes usually comprise some recreational activities such as skipping or ball work, mime for developing the imagination and exercises for each part of the body concentrating on achieving co-ordination, freedom of movement and good posture. Generally, sequences are not taught to juniors because accuracy and hence effectiveness has been found to be better with individual exercises. In a familiar sequence of exercises that the children know by heart, if the movements become indefinite or even incorrect, then they can do more harm that good.

Classes for the two to five year age group were popular in the 1950's and 1960's, before pre-school nurseries were common, giving toddlers a chance to mix with others of their age. The next age group, six to ten years, is the ideal time to correct bad postural habits or to prevent them forming. Marjorie Carpenter opened a junior class in Sutton Coldfield in 1943, and several decades later wrote:

> 'The difficulty of taking children's classes within the League is that of finding enough time in the programme to hold classes for the different age groups. Junior classes are a great joy but they demand from a teacher much more energy than is required for adult classes, and she must have a great love for the type of work and for the children themselves. Quite a number of former Junior League Members are now qualified physical training and dancing teachers and they return to our League classes for pleasure and enjoyment.'

By 1962 Sheila Moore-Tucker's Centre had been running junior classes for twenty two years, and currently had sixty six toddlers, seventy one juniors and thirty three teenagers. That year she wrote:

'I find these classes an absolute joy to teach, I still marvel at the enthusiasm for our work in such young members. I find the babies adorable and though lively, really extraordinarily well behaved. The juniors nearly burst they try so hard. The teenagers are so interested and busy that it never occurs to anyone to misbehave. I also find that we can assist enormously in helping children to gain self confidence. Lots of my old juniors are now married and I have their children in my classes!'

The Sixties was a period of growth with new classes opening. A new Centre in Corringham had one claim to fame, in its junior class was the niece of Eileen Fowler! At that time, Elizabeth Mallett adapted the League's Demonstration Order to exercises for juniors played to nursery rhymes, including Jack and Jill and Baa Baa Black Sheep.

Into the Seventies and Eighties the sizes of classes remained fairly constant. Margaret Maxwell in Kircaldy, had forty five in her babies class and over one hundred from the ages of five to thirteen. Jean Yuill in Campsie, a very small town proud of its League history, established the junior League in 1940 and forty years later the classes were still being run for nearly two hundred children across all the age groups. In Belmont with Shelia Moore-Tucker's class, famous for their Albert Hall appearances, there can be as many as two hundred in the baby class alone, with on average, eighty juniors.

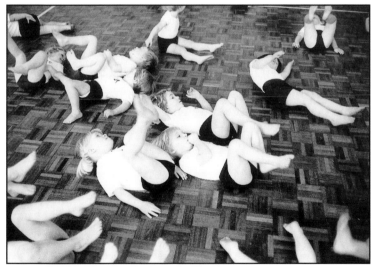

The Belmont Babies

Enthusiasm for junior classes has continued. Chigwell's class started in 1991 and has maintained a steady membership of around twenty ever since, with over two hundred having been members at some time. It is when individual teachers like Alison Sheppard see a need and get so much pleasure from fulfilling it that success is assured. In preparations for most major events, junior items are included and rehearsed with great enthusiasm.

Young teenagers are less easy to attract for a multitude of reasons. The number of alternative activities for them has increased, as has the preference for the most recent trends and fashions. STYLE: Slimming, Toning, Youthful, Lively Exercise was created in 1987 for younger members, to make the exercise experience more attractive to them. One of the prime movers in this venture, Lucy Martin, explained that in the 1930's League members exercised to the pop music of their time and wore a daring uniform and that attracted the young, so why not now? In doing this the League proved that the basic exercise system was adaptable and not reliant on the piano. It also proved a valuable catalyst in establishing other changes; most notably to the idea of a uniform. After just one year STYLE had fourteen classes in Scotland, Lancashire, Wales and Devon, with another ten about to open. Seminars were held around the country to introduce the new techniques to teachers. The first Display where STYLE members presented an item was at the 1990 Diamond Jubilee. The appeal of STYLE classes was so wide that the regular classes were soon exercising to more modern music in brightly coloured leotards, and there became no necessity to hold separate classes.

'Senior' League

League classes have always had their share of senior citizens, and they cope as well with the exercises as any of their juniors. But at the other end of the spectrum there are special problems for those of retirement age who have not done regular exercises throughout their lives. Writing in 1970, Joan Wilder explained the issues:

> 'The problem of adjustment to retirement is recognised as having a very real effect on health, happiness and even length of life. After active years of working life, boredom, loneliness and lack of purpose may depress the spirits and the natural slowing down of physical activity, which occurs as we grow older, can cause minor ailments which may become a handicap to the enjoyment of leisure at the very time of life when we have the opportunity to indulge in it.'

Special classes for older women are a feature of the League, but at retirement age there are men and women who do not feel particularly old and do not want classes with a 'remedial' element. Classes had been held in the 1960's and 1970's at Morley College on Health in Retirement which were open to both sexes. In 1976 there was the first course in a training scheme for teaching the elderly. This was held at St Albans College of Education and was run by League teacher Penny Copple with Joan Wilder as principal tutor. This course later changed its name to EXTEND – Exercise Training for Elderly and Disabled.

The project to develop exercise for the elderly was successfully promoted at national level with a pilot course at St Alban's College in January 1976 and broadcasts by the BBC radio programmes 'Down Your Way ' and 'Woman's Hour' in 1977. 'Age Concern Today' also published an article in their summer edition. By 1978 The President of the British Medical Council was patron, and there was an article about the work of EXTEND published in the medical journal PULSE. Despite all this progress and good work in 1994 its core grant was withdrawn from the Department of Health. The office moved and some staff were made redundant. Yet during that same year over one hundred new EXTEND teachers were trained.

EXTEND has survived but has been constrained in what it can do to respond to perceived need because of limited funds. The training of teachers has continued and there has been a steady growth in the number of classes. By 1986 EXTEND had been going ten years and eighteen courses had produced one hundred and ninety two teachers. Teams of EXTEND members with their tutors have demonstrated to Hospital In-Service Training Days and to numerous exhibitions and conferences including national meetings of the Chest Heart and Stroke Association, and the Registered Nursing Homes Association. In 1989 there were thirty four classes run specifically for senior citizens and the disabled. Between 1994 and 1997 EXTEND doubled in size. The main problems faced by EXTEND are when large numbers of people enquire after classes, when there are none close by.

The success of each of these ventures has been due to the personal commitment and determination of the individuals who set them up. What they show is that the need and demand is there. For the EXTEND classes to develop on a wider scale there would be need for some additional external funding. Then those people who have not been in the League all of their lives, can join in and get more out of life, not just health and well being but fun and friendship.

CHAPTER 12

FIT FOR THE FUTURE

The future is shaped by our decisions today. The decisions made in the past, on teacher training, uniforms, music and exercises, were necessary to enable the organisation to adapt and succeed in a changing and highly competitive environment. The challenge for the future is to ensure that the essence of what makes the League, what it is, remains. When Prunella was asked for her views on the pride that members have in the League's heritage and their concerns about change, she gave a very pragmatic response:

> 'We must make changes in order to make what we know to be a very good product more attractive to prospective members.'

Such clear sighted thinking can only help an organisation find a way forward. Recounting the history of the League shows that the 'very good product' has survived, as have the values that Mary Bagot Stack established, in the 'fitness, fun and friendship for all' ethos that the League still epitomises.

THE CURRENT CONTEXT

Mary Bagot Stack created the League in response to the social needs of the 1930's. In the first decade of the new millennium it is clear that there are still very important social needs that the League can help to fulfil. There has been a tremendous expansion in the choice of different exercise regimes and opportunities to keep fit, as gyms and fitness centres offer a wide range of classes. The fashion recently has been for aerobics with its emphasis on acquiring high levels of cardio-vascular fitness through excessive movement of the legs and arms. However, this only addresses some of the needs of the body and may cause injury. The need to improve fitness, posture and alignment has been better understood by dancers and exercise trends such as pilates, yoga and t'ai chi. Each development takes place within a specific social climate. The 1980's saw a proliferation of exercise tapes and when Jane Fonda launched her version she claimed it was the first to be done to music. The fashion and desire was still to look and feel better but the terminology was very different; not 'grace and expression' but 'energy and endurance'. Increasingly it is being recognised that all those involved in physical activity and sport, as well as the general public, can benefit from the focus on small controlled movements as exemplified by the Bagot Stack system, which continues as The Fitness League.

There has to be something amiss in our more fitness aware society when the generation that has grown up with the diet and exercise industry have also grown more obese. Each New Year sees many people joining gyms. Research reported in the Observer showed that this is an industry worth £1.6 billion. However 75% of people who join gyms stop going within six months. The majority of those who remain members do not do regular exercise, but use other facilities such as the sun beds and saunas. Another report from the University of London's Institute of

Education compared the health of people born in the 1940's to those born in the 1970's. The latter group had greater problems with regard to weight, high blood pressure, asthma and depression. The figures are not much better for the country as a whole: 75% of the population are overweight, and obesity is five times the level it was twenty five years ago. Many people try diets but the central problem for health and well being is that over 60% of people never exercise.

For anyone who does not exercise by the time they reach their thirties they will lose 6oz of muscle mass a year. By the age of forty they will have lost 4lb of muscle which is replaced by fat. This means that metabolism slows down which makes dieting far more difficult. The fact is that as people get older, exercise becomes more important. A recent Mori poll show that for the first time in history in the UK, there are more people over sixty five years of age than under sixteen. The need for the Fitness League is as real as it ever was, and the market is there.

THE LEAGUE MOVES FORWARD

In a recent survey of League members 80% said that the League's system of exercise was more fun and easier to sustain than attending a gym, aerobics or jogging, as well as being cheaper with no special equipment required. It is also far safer. The view of members was that combining effective healthy exercise with movement and music, helped to create a positive mood.

If the 'popular', more image conscious, branches of the fitness industry are not having any effect on the population's general health and well being on any measurable level, then it becomes necessary, not to compete with them but to emphasise how the League is different. As Margaret Peggie wrote in 1995:

> 'It seems obvious now that the continuing health of the League depends on our efforts to demonstrate the difference between what we have to offer people and that which is the province of those we have seen as our competitors. After all, we have come to realise that we are not in the same business of training instructors for aerobics or step exercise classes, which is a very different form of training from the kind of exercise and movement classes which we offer.'

Teachers interviewed each had their own ideas about how to target the market for new League members. The majority realised that women from their mid thirties onwards were more likely to remain members long term. As has been seen this is a huge potential market and one that is growing. The success of EXTEND also shows that there is a demand for the more specialised nature of the League's exercises. The UK has an ageing population and this has led to political concerns about implications for the future cost of health and social care. League members epitomise the reality of the benefits of exercise for their health and well being in older age. MANFIT classes are another innovation that has not yet reached its full potential. Those who have attended classes for a number of years, like their female counterparts have reported on how much better they look and feel.

The young may not be the largest potential source of membership for the League but there is still a very important place for the Junior League. For those teachers who have had success in these areas, the message about health and well being is being transmitted to the young with its longer term benefits for them. Their knowledge and understanding of the League makes them another important source of long term members and teachers.

THE NEXT 75 YEARS

Asking the League 'leaders' what they thought the future held there was guarded optimism. All are sure it will survive, the will is there; it becomes a question of means.

When asked what the prospects were for the League in the 21st Century, Prunella said:

> 'That is hard to answer, it is hard to visualise – I believe we will continue. There is the undeniable fact that it is good to train your body. We offer a system that has sound basic principles. There is a 'holistic' approach present in our work – incorporating dance and expressiveness – which supplies a need that can't easily be satisfied in any other way. I am sure most women appreciate this. The Gym is functional but there is nothing for the mind and spirit. Women will turn to us because of a need to switch off from an increasingly mechanical hi-tech life style and on to something more meaningful and satisfying.'

The Chairman of the Council, Peter Hobden, believes strongly in the future of the League. Since he joined the League in 2003 there have been several new initiatives. In 2004 a Think Tank was established of eight teachers chaired by Sarah Price, to give teachers an opportunity to contribute ideas for the future development of the League. He explained how the management upheavals of the recent past have given the League an insight into what its true needs are. Not only has this been a valuable learning process but the League is now much stronger to face the future. He emphasised that he believed the skills and expertise needed to ensure the League's future could be found from within the League and that he saw part of his role as ensuring that those in the League built up a strong sense of self-belief.

The means to achieve this, then becomes the focal issue. The two key elements remain, of ensuring that there are enough teachers and getting the message to the potential members. Reaching new members can be done either directly or through new forms of collaboration with other bodies and agencies with an interest in health and well being. One interesting new venture was described by Lucy Martin as an 'exciting breakthrough'. The League is embarking on a new course in Lincolnshire where there are very few League teachers. The East Lindsay District Council approached the League as they wanted a 50 plus exercise scheme in all their village halls. This is an important pilot scheme which if successful could be offered to many other local councils. Lucy also explained how the League could benefit from having a higher profile among local health providers, not only in attracting new members but also in attracting more people keen to train as teachers.

Some League teachers are contacting their local Primary Health Care organisations to explain the benefits of League classes in relation to rehabilitation, now that GPs can officially write prescriptions for 'Exercise'. In 2002 Moya Botterill began a pilot study on Exercise on Prescription, in the Dorset area. She knew that the League's system of exercise was better suited to remedial work than most others and it would be a great benefit to individuals, the League and the Health service if League classes could be prescribed and paid for, for those in need. At this stage, such developments tend to be on an informal basis. Getting the necessary information to health care professionals in a more formal way can only help. Over fifty years ago one farsighted SRN wrote to the Nursing Mirror (11th December 1953):

> 'I should like to pay tribute to the work the Women's League of Health and Beauty is doing in the field of preventative medicine. Many post operative and post natal cases are sent to the League by general practitioners; these patients usually continue with the classes long after medical need. The work being done by this small group of hard working teachers, who are doing a great deal towards health education, is still not sufficiently appreciated. I should like to see the name of the nearest League Centre displayed in every health clinic.'

Reaching new members directly should be helped by an increase in the visibility of the League with the 75th anniversary celebrations. The cost of general advertising is prohibitive but when it backs up ongoing publicity or is carefully targeted then it can be effective. Word of mouth as a method of recruitment has served the League very well since the beginning, and should be encouraged so it can continue to do so.

The second aspect of achieving future success, having enough teachers and having a wider geographical spread of classes, is also being addressed by the League. However, establishing a form of 'succession planning' is difficult, when teachers are self employed and cannot be directed to teach in a specific area. A number of the teachers who trained in the late 1960s and 1970s are coming up to, or passing, retirement age and some, quite naturally, wish to reduce their number of classes or to retire altogether. Many continue teaching rather than allow their Centre to close, out of love of the work and loyalty to the League and their members. So the issue of continuing to attract, train and retain teachers is critical.

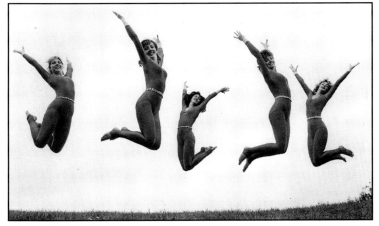

Newly qualified teachers

The systems of Teacher Training within the League have been adapted gradually over the years as a necessary response to changing expectations and social circumstances. The core training has retained its thoroughness and standards, and with increasing recognition by other bodies of the value of this, it is hoped to attract new students. Other forms of assistance are available when a teacher has qualified. They have in the past faced an uphill task to establish new classes which attract sufficient numbers of members to make the enterprise economic. However, when a new teacher takes over an established class, the chances of that class being a long term success are much greater. The new teacher then has the possible problem of facing members who have many more years experience than they have as well as an established set of expectations of what a League teacher should be. When these constraints are seen alongside the opportunities offered elsewhere for exercise teachers to take classes when they have little or no training, it becomes clear just how special League teachers are.

The views expressed by League teachers vary depending upon whether they are new and trying to get established, or whether they have been teaching for many years and have no wish to increase their number of classes or to begin new ones. All of them face the weekly need to attract enough members to at least cover costs, and when the weather is bad or the telly is good, it may be that members do not have the perseverance of the teacher to attend the class. One of the most remarkable factors in this is the great distances that the majority of League teachers are prepared to travel to run a class. It is nothing for many to have a round trip of a hundred miles. On top of the cost of the hall, travel and incidentals such as tapes and licence fees, it is sometimes difficult for teachers to make a reasonable return. When they were asked about this, the replies from well established teachers were very similar. They do it because they love their work and they feel a commitment to their class. To attract more new and younger teachers, the teaching role must offer them an acceptable full or part time income. What both groups of teachers have in common is that they describe the great satisfaction they get from seeing members improve in confidence, movement and co-ordination, and get considerable enjoyment from the class. When they see improvements in the health and well-being of their members, this is their achievement.

The history of the League and the stories of its members and teachers reinforce its tremendous achievements of the last seventy five years. Throughout that time it has met both social and individual needs, and it can continue to do so for another seventy five years and beyond. The benefits of the League exercises are undisputed, and the sum total it has added to human happiness is immeasurable. The League can continue to help to generate this health and well-being on a much wider scale. This is made more difficult because the League, as a not for profit organisation registered as a charity, has limited funds to make its dreams a reality. Very like the time when Mary Bagot Stack had a vision of the future and just £8, a lot of faith, ideals and determination to make it work.

APPENDIX 1

CHRONOLOGY OF KEY EVENTS

1930

League opens in YMCA in Regent St.
Foundation demonstration 12.6.30
100 members, Cockpit, Hyde Park.
Opening of Belfast Centre: Eileen MacMurray.

1931

Membership over 2,000.
First suburban centre at Golders Green.
Second demonstration in Hyde Park.
First Royal Albert Hall display.
Classes moved to the Mortimer Halls.

1932

Seven further centres open at Bromley, Southend, Slough, Bournemouth, Croydon, Birmingham and Glasgow. Followed shortly afterwards by Ayr, Paisley and Edinburgh.
The opening demonstration in Glasgow.
Summer: the third Hyde Park and second Albert Hall displays were held.
Birth of the League magazine, initially called "Mother and Daughter'.
Introduction of a 'uniform'.

1933

League membership reaches 30,000.
First edition of 'Mother and Daughter'.
For 4th year: 500 members in Hyde Park with an audience of 30,000.
Third Albert Hall display.

1934

Membership up to 47,000.
50 students in teacher training.
May: Hyde Park, 1,000 strong, Rally, and Albert Hall. It began with a service at All Souls Church.

1935

January 26th. Death of Mary Bagot Stack: Remembrance Service, All Souls' Church.
League opened in Dublin by Kathleen O'Rourke.
League Centres set up in Australia, Canada & Hong Kong.
Thea Stanley Hughes in Sydney.
Natalie Platner in Toronto.
Kathleen Glover in Hong Kong.
Display at Olympia. 2,500 participants.
64 new centres had opened in Britain.

1936

First Welsh Centre opened at Swansea.
Junior section of League established.
Membership close to 100,000.
Free classes held weekly in deprived areas of Glasgow, Liverpool, Birmingham, Nottingham Brighton, Stepney, Notting Hill, Marylebone.
The League affiliated to the Central Council of Recreative Physical Training.
At Olympia Rally, 5,000. First overseas contingent from Canada.
In memory of Mrs Bagot Stack, a 'Bagot Stack' cot in the Queen's Hospital for Children, from the Memorial Fund.

1937

League introduced to New Zealand by Millicent Ward.
Coronation Pageant Wembley Stadium 12 June: 5,000 participants. Teams from 240 centres: UK, Australia, Canada. Also representatives from Hong Kong, New York and Denmark.
Magazine renamed Health and Beauty.
The Festival of Youth: National Fitness Council. 900 League members attend,

with the King and Queen present.
Prunella invited by Prime Minister Stanley Baldwin to serve on the newly formed National Fitness Council.

1938

Royal Albert Hall display: Margaret Morris Movement & English Folk Dance
Rhythm in Dance and Exercise part of campaign by the National Fitness Council. Queen present.
International Festivals of Physical Culture held in Hamburg, teachers and League team invited.
Classes held at National Federation of Women's Institutes; spreading to over 80 WI branches.
Lord Mayor's Show; 'In Work or Play – Fitness Wins'. With 50 student teachers
League affiliates to the National Council of Women of Great Britain.
17th Dec. First General Meeting of the League under its new formation as a Friendly Society.

1939

Empire Pageant 10th June Wembley Stadium March past: ten foreign and Dominion teams: plus representatives from Canada, Eire, Australia, New York, Hong Kong.
League team of 20 teachers attended the Lingiad Festival in Stockholm.
War declared with Germany.

1940

New centre in Lennoxtown in Stirlingshire.
HQ Revue 'Carry On' held King George's Hall, Russell St. To raise funds for wartime charities.
Prunella takes over as Editor of League magazine.

1941

The League is reconstituted as 'The Women's League of Health and Beauty Limited'.
Mr T. J. M.Macleod became the first Chairman.

1945

London's Thanksgiving Final day display organised by Joan St Lo in Trafalgar Square

1946

The Bagot Stack Health School reopens. Principal Kathleen O'Rourke
First peacetime rally in Hyde Park and Display at Wembley. 1,5000 performers.
League represented at the National Festival of Youth, Empire Pool, Wembley Stadium July.
Teacher's Association formed

1947

First post-war Regional Rally. Birmingham Central Hall.
Two television demonstrations by League teams at Alexandra Palace.

1948

Reopening of Manchester Centre.
Prunella on TV in 'Designed for Women'.
Reunion Display: Scottish members in Glasgow.
Olympic Festival 'Movement is Life' for delegates and Olympic Team.
League classes at Butlin's.
Preston hosts a NW Regional Reunion.
Prunella attends International Congress on Physical Education, Recreation & Rehabilitation in London, 500 delegates from 74 countries.

1949

Reunions in South West and London.

1950

League's change of constitution: formed as non-profit making Association with charity status.

Executive Committee of teachers appointed to advise on day to day management, with Peggy St Lo as Organising Secretary.

20th Anniversary Display & Reunion at Empire Pool Wembley, 1,600 members.

League opens a Centre in British Columbia - Diana Kropinska.

Centre reunions at Derby, Reading area, Norwich and Hastings.

1951

Festival of Britain; League gives demonstrations.

Prunella opens League Centre in South Africa.

League's 21st Anniversary Reunion and Display Royal Albert Hall.

First South African Display in Cape Town.

1952

Edinburgh Festival of Sport: members' displays

League display at South Africa van Reibeek Tercentenary Festival.

1953

Coronation Year Display at Royal Albert Hall. South Africa sends a team. Six items televised.

Birmingham celebrates 21 years with a Reunion and Rally.

1954

21st year of 'Health and Beauty' magazine.

Edinburgh celebrates 20 years, at National Display: Murrayfield Ice rink, Glasgow.

1955

League's Silver Jubilee Display Royal Albert Hall. Dedicated to the memory of the founder.

The Bagot Stack Health School transferred to Morley College, Westminster and renamed Bagot Stack

College. Principle Joan Wilder.

Members contribute to the Festival of Movement and Dance at Wembley.

1956

New League Centre opens in New Zealand: Kay Hudson.

1957

New League Centre in Johannesburg South Africa: Betty Bingham.

Prunella takes over as Principal of the Bagot Stack College from Joan Wilder.

1958

League team at the Festival of Movement and Dance, Wembley.

1959

30th Anniversary Display Royal Albert Hall; many overseas members.

1960

League gives display at the Festival of Movement and Dance Wembley.

1961

Canada's Silver Jubilee.

League Centre opens in Pretoria, South Africa.

Anne Lillis, becomes principal of Bagot Stack College.

1962

League display at the dedication of the new Coventry Cathedral. Local members performed a three part ballet choreographed by Joan & Peggy St Lo.

1963

Royal Albert Hall Demonstration 1st June.

Festival of Movement and Dance, Wembley.

New Centre opens in Salisbury Rhodesia - Daphne Kipps.

1964

Woburn Abbey Displays by invitation of Duke and Duchess of Bedford.

1965

London Centre's 35th Birthday Rally and Reunion. Royal Albert Hall.

1966

Retirement of Deidre Welsh as Musical Director.

1967

League Centre opens in West Vancouver.
Johannesburg's 10th birthday celebrations and first African reunion.
Area Rally for Wessex Centres.
Mr Denis Richards becomes Chairman of League Council.

1968

First Overseas Convention in Toronto.
Woburn Display: invite to Woburn Park.
W Midlands Festival of Movement and Dance. League contributes.

1969

Pioneer Part time Teacher Training Courses: Midlands (Joan Jeffries) and South West (Elizabeth Mallett).
League magazine in new format: 'Poise'.
Vancouver Convention and new Vancouver Centre: Diana Kropinska.

1970

First Associate teachers qualify on part time scheme. Add 1,000 new members.
40th anniversary, weekend Rally in Brighton organised by London Centre, 1,600 attend.
Mr Macleod the League Secretary and Treasurer died and was replaced by Mr H. N. Mussen

1971

Woburn Abbey demonstration 600 members, with Joan Jefferies and Barbara Furniss.
Rhodesian Convention: International Rally, Elizabeth Mallet took a team.
Northern part time training course established Lynn Wallwork and Kirsteen Elmhirst.
First Canadian Teacher Training School: Heather Elliott and Diana Kropinska.

1972

Part time training course established by Pat Rowlandson and Eileen Barnes.
New Centre in Mombasa -Laila Dossa.
New Zealand Convention. Auckland.
National Development Officer: Elizabeth Mallett.
21st Anniversary in Cape Town.

1973

Two further part time teacher training courses in Scotland (Jean Yuill) and in Wales (Gloria Fear).
Exercises for Sport for All, Wembley. 300 League members participate.
Burma Star Association Reunion, Royal Albert Hall - Tricia Hodgkin.
First National Rally in Wales, Cardiff. 1,700 members Gloria Fear.
Rally of Bermuda Health and Beauty Association: Vicki Jensen 170 UK
Keep Fit Association National Festival, Royal Albert Hall. League presents item.
Barbara Furniss appointed Musical Director of the League.

1974

10th Anniversary, Salisbury Rhodesia, S W Training course. Lynn Wallwork.
West Midlands Festival of Movement and Dance. League participates.

1975

45th Birthday celebration. Anniversary Display, Royal Albert Hall. 1,500 performers. Teams from Canada, New Zealand and South Africa.
New North Eastern Training Course: Jean Yuill.

1976

New East Midlands Training Course. Pat Rowlandson.
First course in training for teaching elderly at St Albans College of Education.
Cape Town 25th Birthday celebrations, Prunella visits.
Joan Jefferies appointed Training Officer.

1977

Sport for All weekend organised by the Sports Council. One team marched into the Cockpit, Hyde Park to commemorate the 1930 display.
Vancouver Convention, with visitors from the UK and New Zealand.
Seona Rose succeeds Elizabeth Mallett as National Development Officer.
West Vancouver's 10th birthday.
New Zealand's 40th anniversary.
West Midlands Festival of Movement and Dance. Two League items.

1978

New League Centres open in West Hallam, Droitwich, Norwich, Daventry and Redhill.
Medau Society's 25th Anniversary Royal Albert Hall. Item by 12 League teachers.
City of London Arts Festival: League demonstrations in Paternoster Square.
Johannesburg 21st Birthday.
Retirement of Eileen MacMurray.

1979

Currently 225 League centres running 850 League classes.

1980

Golden Jubilee Celebrations Royal Albert Hall Teams from South Africa, Canada, New Zealand and Eire. 1,150 participants. Receptions at British Columbia House, the South African Embassy & New Zealand House.
Prunella was awarded the OBE in the Queen's Birthday Honours List.

1981

League attends two exhibitions: Active Sports: Birmingham; World of Women 81: Wembley.

1982

Prunella becomes President designate of the League.
Joan and Peggy St Lo retire from teaching after 52 years.
New Courses begin in Scotland, Yorkshire, Home Counties, and Exeter.
Johannesburg and Pretoria 25th and 21st anniversary. Prunella takes a team of teachers.
Thanksgiving Service for the life of Mary Bagot Stack in St Alban's Abbey.
Tricia Hodgkin becomes National Development Officer.

1983

Mary Bagot Stack Centenary celebrations. Classes in Hyde Park. Rally at Albert Hall.
Peggy St Lo retires as Organising Secretary.
Peter Hutton ACIS appointed League Secretary ; new office at 18 Charing Cross Rd.

1984

Liverpool International Garden Festival: Teams from Liverpool, Yorkshire and Midlands contribute, May –September.
First League Class in Holland: Ine Clarke.

1985

CCPR National Festival of Movement and Dance Royal Albert Hall. Two League items.
Committee changes: Margaret Peggie replaces Prunella as Chair of the Training Committee. Barbara Allen replaces Pat Rowlandson as Chair of the Executive Committee.
Stoke Mandeville Hospital: Plaque unveiled commemorating the life and work of Mary Bagot Stack.
International Rugby Festival. Royal Albert Hall. League perform three items.

1986

The League adopts working title of Health and Beauty Exercise.
NDO Tricia Hodgkin retires after introducing regionalisation.
Barbara Furniss retires as Musical Director.
Burma Star Festival Royal Albert Hall with team of Midland members.
League video: 'Doing it in Style' with Lucy Martin and SW teachers.

1987

Death of Vice President Joan St Lo.
League Chairman Denis Richards retires.
New Zealand Golden Jubilee Celebrations. Launch of STYLE. Stretching, Toning, Young Lively Exercise, classes by Lucy Martin.
Celebrating Age: Age Concern, Royal Albert Hall. 90 members, three generations perform.

1988

Norman Abernethy MBE: becomes League Chairman.
Glasgow Garden Festival A team of 80 members perform three times a month.
Head Office moves to the Strand.

1989

Margaret Peggie & Lucy Martin succeed Pat Rowlandson as Training Officers.
Rosemary Barber succeeds Barbara Allen as Executive Chairman, and appointed as Liaison Officer for Teachers – a new post.

1990

Diamond Jubilee Celebrations Royal Albert Hall. Participants from New Zealand, Canada, South Africa, Zimbabwe, Pakistan, Ireland, Holland.
Message from her Majesty the Queen.
Presentations to 75 members who joined before 1935.

1991

Reunion for pre-war teachers.12 still teaching! Margaret Peggie: Vice Chairman of the Movement & Dance Division & on the Executive of the CCPR (Central Council of Physical Recreation.)
Cape Town 40th anniversary Rally.

1992

National Rally and Inter-Centre Competition Fairfield Hall Croydon. 17 Centres compete.
Ideal Homes Exhibition. League item.
Training Committee modifies the Bagot Stack Demonstration Order which has stood since 1930.

1993

Vancouver Celebrates 25th birthday. Many UK members attend.

1994

League Fairfield Festival in Croydon, 1,200 members 13 items.
Diamond Jubilee of the League of Health, Ireland. Tribute to Isolde McCullagh, the Principal.
'Ballroom Blitz' Royal Albert Hall. League perform two displays.
Dance World Exhibition Barbican,

teachers and members perform three items
League moves to offices in Chertsey.
Peter Hutton retires as chair but remains as Company Secretary. Administration taken over by teachers: Val Augustine - Administration Officer, Rosemary Barber - Internal Liaison, Margaret Peggie - External Liaison, Lucy Martin continues as Training Officer.
Kathleen Ward retires, aged 90, after 60 years of teaching.

1995

Leagues 65th Anniversary; Royal Albert Hall.
Dance World show at Olympia.
National Festival of Movement and Dance at Royal Albert Hall.
MANFIT Commenced.
Mr Leslie Cond new Council chairman.

1997

Harrogate Spa Spectacular.
New Zealand's 60th Birthday. celebrations. 100 members from UK and S Africa attended.

1999

Change of name to The Fitness League.
Newly appointed full time manager.
Executive Committee renamed Liaison Committee.
New Council Chairman Neil Phillips.

2000

15th April 70th Birthday held at the Royal Albert Hall.
Dancefest 2000 at Royal Albert Hall.
Cape Town's 50th Anniversary.
Executive/Liaison Committee dissolved Liaison Officer post discontinued.

2001

Peggy St Lo died in January, a Thanksgiving Service in September.
Magazine renamed 'Fitness'.
Full time manager post replaced by leadership under the Management Team.

2002

Inscribed bench in memory of the St Lo sisters placed in Hyde Park.

2003

League at the National Festival at the Chester Gateway Theatre.
New Chairman of the Council Peter Hobden.
Informal Exercise, Movement and Dance Partnership, between The Fitness League, the Keep Fit Association, Medau, Margaret Morris Movement and the English Folk Dance Society.

2004

Prunella's 90th Birthday: celebrated at the Teacher's Course in Torquay. Presented with a Book of Memories given by Teachers Association, compiled by Lynne Berry.
Marjorie Duncombe's 100th birthday.
Ireland's 70th Anniversary with Display, classes and dinner in Dublin.
Think Tank formed.

2005

75th Anniversary, April 16th at the Royal Albert Hall.

Appendix 2

The Exercises

With the creation of the Women's League of Health and Beauty in 1930, the Bagot Stack exercise system became more standardised so that the same exercises and sequences were taught in each class. Mary Bagot Stack encouraged members to do one class a week and to exercise for fifteen minutes each day. Her slogan for healthy slimness was 'stretch and swing'. It was also emphasised that no effective stretching was possible until the joints were loosened, particularly those of the spine. Each exercise had its own sequence of movements and a title. For example 'The Elephant' required the student to be on all fours with the knees and elbows perfectly straight and the palms of the hands flat on the ground; this was for stretching and loosening the spine – all important for good posture. As exercise sequences became standardised they were put to music so that they were easier to learn. Mary compared this to learning poetry by heart. Her exercises would be physical poetry.

The main tenet of the Bagot Stack system was Central Control, wherein a steady centre for the body is made by the lower back and abdomen being drawn strongly towards each other. Other important aspects included elastic breathing, relaxation, mobilisation and strengthening, and heel stretching. Classes consisted of rhythmical, continuous and co-ordinated movements set to music and were originally graduated into elementary, intermediate and advanced classes so that no one was over stretched. Above all the sessions were meant to be fun. In a newspaper interview, Prunella describes the League as 'teaching women to laugh their way to health'. Enjoyment of exercise was fundamental to Mary Bagot Stack's philosophy, as she understood the extent to which joy and happiness could enhance general well being. This was not necessarily a supposition that was held by other physical trainers either then or today!

Over the following decades the exercise routines that Mary had created were continually developed to incorporate current health and medical knowledge. At all times, though, they had to adhere to Mary's principles that they be safe and effective. The League's system of exercise has grown and developed in line with improved medical knowledge, with some routines being replaced with new ones. The therapeutic foundation of the League's exercises remains as valid today as it ever was. Their booklet on exercises for before and after operations, designed for anyone who is confined to bed for a period of time, has been approved by the National Osteoporosis Society and the Breast Care and Mastectomy Association of GB.

The League has developed a low impact exercise system with 'core stability', which uses small controlled movements to stabilise the torso, as an essential precursor to safe, effective exercise. Earlier, this was referred to as 'the lower back and abdomen being pulled strongly together'. This small movement can be carried out whilst in many positions, standing, lying or sitting, and in each it serves to strengthen the deepest layer of transverse abdominal muscle. At the same time it helps to stabilise the spine. In the days before occupations and life in general became so sedentary, these muscles were used to a far greater extent. As people move around less, flexibility decreases and this puts a strain on the lower back. The effect of having strong transverse abdominal muscles acts like a corset taking the pressure off the back and pulling the other abdominal muscles into place. This 'central control' was the starting point, in the exercise technique. A further benefit was improved posture.

The human torso can be described as having two 'layers' of muscles, the 'inner' and the 'outer'. The inner comprise the transverse abdominal muscles, the diaphragm and the muscles of the pelvis floor. Effective functioning of these is considered essential in preventing back injury and ensuring optimal performance. The outer layer comprises the other abdominal muscles as well as the muscles of the back, pelvis and hip which working together contribute to the stabilisation of the pelvic girdle and spine, as movement occurs. Exercises which strengthen and tone both these sets of muscles form an integral part to any League class. The movements required are small and subtle but if practiced regularly help to prevent back pain, improve posture and flatten stomachs. The physical benefits include reduced joint problems, increased muscular strength and greater flexibility of joints with improved co-ordination and stability.

Participation in classes helps to decrease stress, increase energy levels and is invariably described as fun. It is unlikely ever to result in strain as the movements are gentle and remain within the individual's capabilities. Although it is not designed to burn calories, it will improve body shape and it can help to tone the body of anyone who is on a diet and losing weight. This technique is suitable for anyone, and has been particularly designed to ensure that everyone can gain optimum benefit from any exercise they do.